T0198266

A Surgeon's Guide to Sarcomas and Other Soft Tissue Tumors

Editor

JOHN M. KANE III

SURGICAL CLINICS
OF NORTH AMERICA

www.surgical.theclinics.com

Consulting Editor
RONALD F. MARTIN

August 2022 • Volume 102 • Number 4

ELSEVIER

1600 John F. Kennedy Boulevard ● Suite 1800 ● Philadelphia, Pennsylvania, 19103-2899

http://www.surgical.theclinics.com

SURGICAL CLINICS OF NORTH AMERICA Volume 102, Number 4
August 2022 ISSN 0039–6109, ISBN-13: 978-0-323-91961-6

Editor: John Vassallo, j.vassallo@elsevier.com

Developmental Editor: Arlene Campos

Surgical Clinics of North America (ISSN 0039–6109) is published bimonthly by Elsevier Inc., 360 Park Avenue South, New York, NY 10010-1710. Months of publication are February, April, June, August, October, and December. Business and Editorial Offices: 1600 John F. Kennedy Blvd., Suite 1800, Philadelphia, PA 19103-2899. Periodicals postage paid at New York, NY and additional mailing offices. Subscription prices are $456.00 per year for US individuals, $1240.00 per year for US institutions, $100.00 per year for US & Canadian students and residents, $547.00 per year for Canadian individuals, $1283.00 per year for Canadian institutions, $552.00 for international individuals, $1283.00 per year for international institutions and $250.00 per year for foreign students/residents. To receive student/resident rate, orders must be accompanied by name of affiliated institution, date of term, and the *signature* of program/residency coordinator on institution letterhead. Orders will be billed at individual rate until proof of status is received. Foreign air speed delivery is included in all *Clinics* subscription prices. All prices are subject to change without notice. POSTMASTER: Send address changes to *Surgical Clinics*, Elsevier Health Sciences Division, Subscription Customer Service, 3251 Riverport Lane, Maryland Heights, MO 63043. **Customer Service (orders, claims, online, change of address): Telephone: 1-800-654-2452 (U.S. and Canada); 314-447-8871 (outside U.S. and Canada). Fax: 314-447-8029. E-mail: journalscustomerservice-usa@elsevier.com (for print support); journalsonlinesupport-usa@elsevier.com (for online support).**

Reprints. For copies of 100 or more, of articles in this publication, please contact the Commercial Reprints Department, Elsevier Inc., 360 Park Avenue South, New York, New York 10010-1710. Tel. 212-633-3874, Fax: 212-633-3820, E-mail: reprints@elsevier.com.

Surgical Clinics of North America is also published in Spanish by McGraw-Hill Interamericana Editores S.A., P.O. Box 5-237 06500 Mexico D.F. Mexico; and in Portuguese by Interlivros Edicoes Ltda., Rua Comandante Coelho 1085, CEP 21250, Rio de Janeiro, Brazil; and in Greek by Paschalidis Medical Publications, Athens Greece.

Surgical Clinics of North America is covered in *MEDLINE/PubMed (Index Medicus), EMBASE/Excerpta Medica, Current Contents/Clinical Medicine, Current Contents/Life Sciences, Science Citation Index,* and *ISI/BIOMED.*

Contributors

CONSULTING EDITOR

RONALD F. MARTIN, MD, FACS
Colonel (Retired), United States Army, Department of General Surgery, Pullman Surgical Associates, Pullman Regional Hospital and Clinic Network, Pullman, Washington

EDITOR

JOHN M. KANE III, MD
Chair, Department of Surgical Oncology, Chief of the Melanoma/Sarcoma Service, Roswell Park Comprehensive Cancer Center, Buffalo, New York

AUTHORS

RUSSELL S. BERMAN, MD
Vice Chair for Surgical Education and Faculty Affairs, Chief Division of Surgical Oncology, Director Surgical Residency, Professor of Surgery, NYU Grossman School of Medicine, New York, New York

KENNETH CARDONA, MD, FACS
Patricia R. Reynolds Professor of Sarcoma, Winship Cancer Institute, Division of Surgical Oncology, Department of Surgery, Emory University, Atlanta, Georgia

ILARIA CATUREGLI, MD
Department of Surgery, Brigham and Women's Hospital, Harvard Medical School, Boston, Massachusetts

MICHAEL R. CLAY, MD
Department of Pathology, University of Colorado, Aurora, Colorado

AIMEE M. CRAGO, MD, PhD, FACS
Associate Attending Surgeon, Gastric and Mixed Tumor Service, Department of Surgery, Memorial Sloan Kettering Cancer Center, New York, New York

JEFFREY M. FARMA, MD, FACS
Fox Chase Cancer Center, Philadelphia, Pennsylvania

VALERIE P. GRIGNOL, MD
Associate Professor of Surgery, Division of Surgical Oncology, The Ohio State University Wexner Medical Center, The James Cancer Hospital and Solove Research Institute, Columbus, Ohio

MARK HENNON, MD, FACS
Associate Professor of Oncology, Associate Professor of Surgery, Department of Thoracic Surgery, Roswell Park Comprehensive Cancer Center, Department of Surgery, Jacobs School of Medicine, State University of New York at Buffalo, Buffalo, New York

JOHN M. KANE III, MD
Chair, Department of Surgical Oncology, Chief of the Melanoma/Sarcoma Service, Roswell Park Comprehensive Cancer Center, Buffalo, New York

GIORGOS C. KARAKOUSIS, MD
Associate Professor of Surgery, Department of Endocrine and Oncologic Surgery, Hospital of the University of Pennsylvania, Department of Surgery, Philadelphia, Pennsylvania

SARA KRYEZIU, MD
Resident, Department of General Surgery, NYU Grossman School of Medicine, New York, New York

ANN Y. LEE, MD
Assistant Professor, Department of Surgery, Associate Program Director Surgical Residency, NYU Grossman School of Medicine, New York, New York

ROBERT F. LOHMAN, MD, MBA
Associate Professor of Oncology, Department of Plastic and Reconstructive Surgery, Roswell Park Comprehensive Cancer Center, Buffalo, New York

ALEXANDRA G. LOPEZ-AGUIAR, MD, MS
Surgical Oncology Fellow, Division of Surgical Oncology, The Ohio State University Wexner Medical Center, The James Cancer Hospital and Solove Research Institute, Columbus, Ohio

GARY N. MANN, MD
Associate Professor of Oncology, Department of Surgical Oncology, Roswell Park Comprehensive Cancer Center, Buffalo, New York

MARTIN M. McCARTER, MD
Department of Surgery, University of Colorado, Aurora, Colorado

ANKIT PATEL, MD
Surgical Oncology Fellow, Department of Surgical Oncology, Roswell Park Comprehensive Cancer Center, Buffalo, New York

ANDREA S. PORPIGLIA, MD, FACS
Fox Chase Cancer Center, Philadelphia, Pennsylvania

KATHERINE PRENDERGAST, MD
Research Fellow, Sarcoma Biology Laboratory, Memorial Sloan Kettering Cancer Center, New York, New York

CHANDRAJIT P. RAUT, MD, MSc, FACS, FSSO
Chief, Division of Surgical Oncology, Department of Surgery, Brigham and Women's Hospital, Surgery Director, Center for Sarcoma and Bone Oncology, Dana-Farber Cancer Institute, Professor of Surgery, Harvard Medical School, Boston, Massachusetts

KILIAN E. SALERNO, MD
Associate Research Physician, Staff Clinician, Clinical Director, Radiation Oncology Branch, National Cancer Institute, National Institutes of Health, Bethesda, Maryland

CIMARRON E. SHARON, MD
Hospital of the University of Pennsylvania, Department of Surgery, Philadelphia, Pennsylvania

CAMILLE L. STEWART, MD
Department of Surgery, University of Colorado, Aurora, Colorado

ZACHARY E. STILES, DO, MS
Surgical Oncology Fellow, Department of Surgical Oncology, Roswell Park Comprehensive Cancer Center, Buffalo, New York

RICHARD J. STRAKER III, MD
Hospital of the University of Pennsylvania, Department of Surgery, Philadelphia, Pennsylvania

MICHAEL K. TURGEON, MD
Katz Foundation Research Fellow, Winship Cancer Institute, Division of Surgical Oncology, Department of Surgery, Emory University, Atlanta, Georgia

GERARDO A. VITIELLO, MD
Department of Surgery, Division of Surgical Oncology, NYU Langone Health, CGSO Fellow, Memorial Sloan Kettering Cancer Center, New York, New York

ELAINE T. Vo, MD
Fox Chase Cancer Center, Philadelphia, Pennsylvania

ELLIOTT J. YEE, MD
Department of Surgery, University of Colorado, Aurora, Colorado

Contents

Foreword: Sarcoma   xiii

Ronald F. Martin

Preface: The Suspicious Soft Tissue Mass   xvii

John M. Kane III

The Implications of an Unplanned Sarcoma Excision (the "Whoops" Operation)   529

Valerie P. Grignol and Alexandra G. Lopez-Aguiar

In this review, the risk factors of an unplanned excision of soft-tissue sarcoma and the implications of non-oncologic resection are discussed. Although soft-tissue sarcoma remains a rare disease, many studies have shown the deleterious effects of unplanned excision, including decreased recurrence-free survival and increased morbidity. Once discovered, sarcomas should be referred to expert centers for further management, which often entails re-excision, radiation, and/or chemotherapy treatment. Although much still needs to be learned about this complex disease, a multidisciplinary approach including surgeons, medical oncologists, radiologists, and pathologists is paramount to its successful treatment.

The Role of Imaging in Soft Tissue Sarcoma Diagnosis and Management   539

Cimarron E. Sharon, Richard J. Straker III, and Giorgos C. Karakousis

The differential diagnosis of a soft tissue mass is broad, and an appropriate imaging workup is crucial to accurate identification. Additionally, imaging plays a critical role in soft tissue sarcoma (STS) staging and monitoring for disease progression. In this article, we discuss the different imaging modalities and their utility in the workup and surveillance of STS.

Wide Resection of Extremity/Truncal Soft Tissue Sarcomas   551

Ankit Patel and John M. Kane III

The potentially curative treatment of sarcoma is negative margin wide resection, the clinical tumor with an en bloc margin of surrounding tissue potentially contains microscopic tumor. Planned margins should be 1 to 2 cm but can be less for oncologically equivalent barrier tissues or to preserve an adjacent critical structure. Tumor spillage should be avoided. The role of radiation and/or chemotherapy should be discussed before surgery, as there are potential benefits to preoperative administration. An isolated local recurrence is potentially curable. Amputation is rarely necessary and should only be pursued after other limb salvage treatment options have been considered.

Radiation Therapy for Soft Tissue Sarcoma: Indications, Timing, Benefits, and
Consequences   567

Kilian E. Salerno

Radiation therapy is an integral component of local management with oncologic resection for soft tissue sarcoma. In patients at an increased risk or local recurrence, radiotherapy is indicated to improve local control. Sequencing of radiotherapy and resection should be determined by multidisciplinary input before treatment initiation. For most patients, preoperative delivery of radiation therapy is preferred. In patients initially thought to be at low risk for local recurrence and found to have unexpected adverse pathologic features at resection, postoperative radiation therapy is indicated. The use of radiation therapy for retroperitoneal sarcoma is controversial; when used, preoperative delivery of radiation is recommended.

Plastic Surgery Reconstruction of Sarcoma Resection Defects: Form and Function   583

Zachary E. Stiles, Robert F. Lohman, and Gary N. Mann

Surgical wide resection is the mainstay of treatment of sarcomas, but the advent of multimodality therapy has improved outcomes and the rates of limb-sparing resection. Often, wounds are unable to be closed primarily and require plastic surgical reconstruction. Following adequate oncologic resection, reconstruction should focus on maintaining functional and esthetic outcomes with minimal postoperative complications. Reconstruction methods range from simple techniques such as skin grafting and local rotational flaps all the way to more complex procedures such as free flaps. The reconstructive surgeon is an integral member of the multidisciplinary team and should be actively involved in treatment planning.

Retroperitoneal Sarcomas: Histology Is Everything   601

Michael K. Turgeon and Kenneth Cardona

Retroperitoneal sarcomas (RPS) are a rare subset of soft tissue sarcoma that are composed of only a few histologic subtypes, each with a distinct tumor biology, clinical presentation, preferred treatment strategy, recurrence risk, and surveillance plan. In the modern era of precision medicine, our understanding of the implications of subtype tumor biology and anatomic location has led to a more nuanced, histology-specific approach to therapy, including surgery, neoadjuvant radiation therapy, and/or chemotherapy. This article provides a summary of recent updates to the management of RPS.

Sarcoma Pulmonary Metastatic Disease: Still a Chance for Cure   615

Mark Hennon

Tumors of soft tissue origin are not common but are increasing in incidence. Given the rare and heterogeneous nature of the disease, deciding on an effective treatment approach to the patient can be challenging. Approximately 20-50% of patients with sarcoma will develop metastases to the lung via hematogenous spread. Despite improvements in systemic therapy options for patients with metastatic disease to the lung, surgical resection of metastases is often the preferred option in patients who are safe surgical candidates. Clearance of metastatic disease with surgical resection has been proven to be cost-effective and can improve chances for long term survival. Deciding on who may benefit from surgical resection is best achieved in a multidisciplinary setting.

Gastrointestinal Stromal Tumors and the General Surgeon   625

Ilaria Caturegli and Chandrajit P. Raut

Gastrointestinal stromal tumors (GISTs) are rare malignancies of the gastrointestinal tract but are the most common sarcoma. This review covers aspects of the care of patients with GIST relevant to surgeons. In particular, management of sub-2 cm GISTs, the utility of neoadjuvant and adjuvant therapy for primary GISTs, and indications for surgery in the setting of metastatic disease are discussed.

Lipoma and Its Doppelganger: The Atypical Lipomatous Tumor/Well-Differentiated Liposarcoma   637

Elliott J. Yee, Camille L. Stewart, Michael R. Clay, and Martin M. McCarter

Lipomatous tumors are among the most common soft tissue lesions encountered by the general surgeon. Shared history and clinical presentation make differentiation between benign lipomas and low-grade liposarcomas a diagnostic dilemma. This article reviews the epidemiology, clinical history, diagnostic workup, management, natural history, and surveillance of benign lipomas and atypical lipomatous tumors/well-differentiated liposarcomas. Although it is important that aggressive, potentially malignant atypical lipomatous tumors and liposarcomas be managed in a multidisciplinary, preferably high-volume setting, it is equally as important for the nonspecialist general surgeon to be familiar with lipoma and its doppelganger—the well-differentiated liposarcoma.

Dermatofibrosarcoma Protuberans: What Is This?   657

Gerardo A. Vitiello, Ann Y. Lee, and Russell S. Berman

Dermatofibrosarcoma protuberans (DFSP) is a rare, locally aggressive dermal-based sarcoma. Metastatic potential is extremely low, primarily in the setting of fibrosarcomatous transformation. DFSP is characterized by a t(17;22) (q22;q13) translocation that results in active PDGFB signaling. Surgical resection with negative margins (typically including the underlying fascia) is the potentially curative treatment. Delayed wound closure should be considered for cases requiring extensive resection or tissue rearrangement. Tyrosine kinase inhibitors, such as imatinib, have shown response rates of 50% to 60% in patients with locally advanced or metastatic disease. Radiation can be useful for residual or recurrent diseases.

The Evolving Management of Desmoid Fibromatosis   667

Katherine Prendergast, Sara Kryeziu, and Aimee M. Crago

Desmoid fibromatosis is a rare disease caused by genetic alterations that activate β-catenin. The tumors were previously treated with aggressive surgeries but do not metastasize and may regress spontaneously. For these reasons, in the absence of symptoms and when growth would not induce significant complications, active observation is considered first-line therapy. When intervention is required, surgery can be considered based on anatomy and risk of postoperative recurrence, but increasingly nonoperative therapies such as liposomal doxorubicin or sorafenib are prescribed. Cryoablation, chemoembolization, and high-intensity focused ultrasound can also be used to obtain local control in selected patients.

Benign Neurogenic Tumors   679

Jeffrey M. Farma, Andrea S. Porpiglia, and Elaine T. Vo

Neurogenic tumors arise from cells of the nervous system. These tumors can be found anywhere along the distribution of the sympathetic and parasympathetic nervous system and are categorized based on cell of origin: ganglion cell, paraganglion cell, and nerve sheath cells. Ganglion cell-derived tumors include neuroblastomas, ganglioneuroblastomas, and ganglioneuromas. Paraganglion cell-derived tumors include paragangliomas and pheochromocytomas. Nerve sheath cell-derived tumors include schwannomas (neurilemmomas), neurofibromas, and neurofibromatosis. Most of these are benign; however, they can cause local compressive symptoms. Surgery is the mainstay of treatment, if clinically indicated. Nonetheless, a thorough preoperative workup is essential, especially for catecholamine-secreting tumors.

SURGICAL CLINICS
OF NORTH AMERICA

FORTHCOMING ISSUES

OCTOBER 2022
Pediatric Surgery
John D. Horton, *Editor*

DECEMBER 2022
Management of Benign Breast Disease
Melissa Kaptanian, *Editor*

FEBRUARY 2023
Breast Cancer Management
Anna S. Seydel and Lee G. Wilke, *Editors*

RECENT ISSUES

JUNE 2022
Cardiothoracic Surgery
Daniel G. Cuadrado, *Editor*

APRIL 2022
Head and Neck Surgery
Brian J. Mitchell and Kyle Tubbs, *Editors*

FEBRUARY 2022
Surgical Critical Care
Brett H. Waibel, *Editor*

SERIES OF RELATED INTEREST

Advances in Surgery
https://www.advancessurgery.com/
Surgical Oncology Clinics
https://www.surgonc.theclinics.com/
Thoracic Surgery Clinics
http://www.thoracic.theclinics.com/

THE CLINICS ARE AVAILABLE ONLINE!
Access your subscription at:
www.theclinics.com

Foreword

Sarcoma

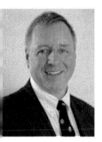

Ronald F. Martin,
MD, FACS
Consulting Editor

It has been said that medicine is an unusual industry in that its goal is to make itself obsolete. That may be the case in some circumstances, but I would say that it not likely to happen any time soon. In some areas of medicine, we may be closer to reducing the need for our services, while in other areas we are certainly generating increased demand for services. Also, given that health care as economic entity writ large represents approximately one-fifth of the US gross domestic product, there are substantial forces at play that must assure that any downward pressure on the need for medical care will be incremental at best.

Acknowledging the above, there is every reason to believe that even if the overall demand for medical care doesn't change dramatically, the ways by which medical care is delivered will be much more amenable to shifts. Perhaps in no aspect of health care is this "internal shifting" more likely to happen than in the general field of oncology.

For much of recorded history, our options to treat cancer were fairly confined to extirpation. We have only had a basic accurate understanding of DNA for less than 80 years, and the improvements on understanding of cellular function, cell-cycle control, and neoplastic biology we have today are largely a function of knowledge gained over the last quarter century.

The use of knives and string (plus videoscopes and robots) to manage cancer has advanced over the last 50 years but at paces that are far outmatched by nonoperative means over the same timeframe. We have moved far past limited cytotoxic chemotherapy to biomodulation and have made some inroads into gene-manipulation for many neoplastic conditions—but not all. Advances in local control with radiation and other local therapies have been substantial as well. The days of operative management being the main focus of attention with all other therapeutic modalities in minor support roles are pretty well behind us now.

Some basic tenets of oncologic care from the early days remain true and likely will for some time. One still needs to be able to correctly diagnose neoplasms, stage

Surg Clin N Am 102 (2022) xiii–xv
https://doi.org/10.1016/j.suc.2022.05.006
0039-6109/22/© 2022 Published by Elsevier Inc.

neoplastic disease, and develop an accurate understanding and prediction of future clinical course to know how to treat the patient. How we evaluate the patient with known or potential cancer has and will continue to evolve and, it is hoped, improve.

A respected mentor to me and many, many others, Dr Blake Cady, once stated in his presidential address to the Society for Surgical Oncology that, as regards cancer, "Biology is king, patient selection is queen, and all the techniques are the princes and princesses of the realm." The use of monarchy and gender-related terms put aside, the general concept is every bit as true today as when he first said it. Our goal must *always* be to understand the biology of the process we are faced with. That coupled with an understanding of which tools to use and how to combine them is how we will achieve maximum therapeutic effect with minimum harm.

This issue of the *Surgical Clinics* on Sarcoma developed by Dr Kane and his colleagues delves into a particularly challenging area of oncologic care. The biology of soft tissue tumors is complex. The anatomic distribution of these tumors frequently puts them in places where local control either by operative means or by other means of directed therapy is constrained by technical limitations and critical adjacent structures. Furthermore, the skill sets required—particularly operative skills—are not easily "cross-trained" for with other operative concerns. If one has performed a high volume of small bowel anastomoses, it should not be too hard to perform a colonic anastomosis. Even if one has done thousands of bowel resections, that may not train one too well to rummage about the retroperitoneum or near the critical neurovascular structures in an extremity.

The collection of articles in this issue should give the reader a sound foundation for the principles of diagnosing, assessing, and treatment options for soft tissue tumors. I think the reader will not only find useful information for the treatment of patients with these problems but also get excellent advice about how to avoid missteps along the way, most importantly, in the early portion of the process when small mistakes can have large long-term consequences.

The principle of "First, do no harm" is well ingrained in us as physicians—it is also wrong, or at least misleading. More accurately, we must strive for no *net harm*. More often than not, when we do something for someone, we also do something to someone. The mere act of operating upon a patient inflicts some harm for which the benefit must justify the action. Failure to do things for people can be as harmful or worse as well.

Neither nihilism nor zealotry is warranted in the care of patients—especially patients who suffer from cancer. We cannot, or at least should not, hate disease more than we love patients. Our ability to distinguish the correct path is to carefully remember what Dr Cady tried to teach us. We must understand the biology of the disease in question. We must select our patients carefully, fully applying the patients' desires in that selection (in my opinion). Last, we must understand the techniques and treatment options in general but also in our own hands. Being honest with our patients and with ourselves is the only way to serve properly those who count on us.

Ronald F. Martin, MD, FACS
Colonel (retired), United States Army Reserve
Department of General Surgery
Pullman Surgical Associates
Pullman Regional Hospital and Clinic Network
825 Southeast Bishop Boulevard, Suite 130
Pullman, WA 99163, USA

E-mail address:
rfmcescna@gmail.com

Preface

The Suspicious Soft Tissue Mass

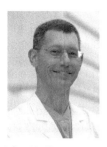

John M. Kane III, MD
Editor

Surgeons are frequently referred patients for the evaluation of a soft tissue mass. Given that "common things occur commonly," the majority will be benign entities such as a lipoma, epidermal inclusion cyst, hematoma, abscess, ganglion cyst, and such. Surgical excision is often the definitive treatment. However, when the mass is a sarcoma or some other soft tissue neoplasm, surgery as the initial treatment can be suboptimal. Consequently, when the clinical history or physical examination does not fit with a more common benign process, one should pause to consider further workup of the mass prior to surgery. Features associated with a higher risk of a mass being a sarcoma include size greater than 5 cm, deep to the muscular fascia, and lower-extremity anatomic location. Rapid enlargement as reported by the patient would also be atypical for a lipoma or other benign entities. In this situation, obtaining high-quality 3-dimensional imaging and considering image-guided core needle biopsies if there are suspicious radiographic features before proceeding to the operating room would be the ideal approach.

The purpose of this issue is to provide a general overview of the current management of soft tissue sarcomas as well as some other more common soft tissue tumors (dermatofibrosarcoma protuberans, desmoid, and benign neurogenic tumors). For sarcomas, a preoperative diagnosis is critical for determining the sequencing of multimodality therapy (radiation, chemotherapy), the planned extent of the wide resection, and reconstruction options (including upfront involvement of plastic surgery). Not only does unplanned excision of a soft tissue sarcoma preclude the ability to administer preoperative radiation or neoadjuvant chemotherapy but also seeding of the surgical site with microscopic sarcoma cells from tumor spillage can significantly decrease the likelihood of obtaining long-term local control. In the modern era, the initial management of some benign tumors, such as desmoids and neurogenic tumors, is often nonsurgical.

Surg Clin N Am 102 (2022) xvii–xviii
https://doi.org/10.1016/j.suc.2022.05.003
0039-6109/22/© 2022 Published by Elsevier Inc.

surgical.theclinics.com

As soft tissue sarcomas are rare, one should not be scared into approaching every single soft tissue mass encountered in practice as if it could be a sarcoma. Rather, the intent is to create a broader differential diagnosis that includes a sarcoma and other soft tissue masses when the clinical presentation is not typical for a benign process. To take the advice from the world of carpentry (another profession that combines judgment and craftsmanship), "measure twice, cut once."

John M. Kane III, MD
Department of Surgical Oncology
Roswell Park Comprehensive Cancer Center
Elm and Carlton Streets
Buffalo, NY 14263, USA

E-mail address:
john.kane@roswellpark.org

The Implications of an Unplanned Sarcoma Excision (the "Whoops" Operation)

Valerie P. Grignol, MD*, Alexandra G. Lopez-Aguiar, MD, MS

KEYWORDS

- Unplanned excision • Extremity soft-tissue sarcoma • Re-excision
- Specialty center

KEY POINTS

- Soft-tissue masses greater than 5 cm, particularly those in the deep compartments, should undergo imaging and core needle biopsy before resection.
- The "whoops" operation is associated with increased local disease recurrence rates.
- After an unplanned excision, salvage wide resection by a sarcoma specialist is indicated.
- Management of soft-tissue sarcomas is best performed at a high-volume institution with a multidisciplinary expert team.

Soft-tissue sarcomas (STSs) are a group of both rare and heterogeneous malignancies that comprise about 1% of all adult cancers.[1] With over 100 histologic subtypes, STS frequently requires complex multidisciplinary management that involves a team of specialized surgeons, radiologists, medical oncologists, and pathologists (**Table 1**).[1] The cornerstone of the curative oncologic treatment of STS is an optimal en bloc surgical resection with a negative margin.2 Although clinical practice guidelines recommend the management of sarcomas at high-volume centers with expertise in the field, due to their rarity, these tumors are frequently and inadvertently misdiagnosed.[2]As such, many patients undergo inadequate diagnostic procedures or lack preoperative imaging before resection. This leads to the entity known as the "Whoops" operation or an unplanned sarcoma excision that has multiple implications.

CLINICAL PRESENTATION OF SOFT-TISSUE SARCOMA

The common presentation of STS is one of a patient with a slowly enlarging soft-tissue lesion, sometimes noticed after a trauma.[3]Although STS can arise anywhere

Division of Surgical Oncology, The Ohio State University Wexner Medical Center, James Cancer Hospital and Solove Research, 460 West 10th Avenue, Columbus, OH 43210, USA
* Corresponding author.
E-mail address: Valerie.Grignol@osumc.edu

Surg Clin N Am 102 (2022) 529–538
https://doi.org/10.1016/j.suc.2022.04.002
0039-6109/22/© 2022 Elsevier Inc. All rights reserved.
surgical.theclinics.com

Table 1 Common soft-tissue sarcoma histologic subtypes[1]	
Other	38%
Leiomyosarcoma	12%
Undifferentiated pleomorphic sarcoma	11%
GIST	7%
Dedifferentiated liposarcoma	6%
Well-differentiated liposarcoma	6%
Desmoid	5%
Angiosarcoma	3%
Chondrosarcoma	3%
Ewing's sarcoma	3%
Myxofibrosarcoma	3%
Synovial sarcoma	3%

throughout the body, about 40% to 50% occur in the extremities (**Fig. 1**).[4,5] There are multiple other diagnoses that are on the clinician's differential when examining a patient with a soft-tissue mass. These include benign lesions (lipomas, subcutaneous cysts, and hematoma) and malignancies (melanoma or lymphoma).[6] Given the much higher frequency of nonmalignant soft-tissue masses, up to 50% of patients with STS undergo an unplanned, non-oncologic excision for a mass initially believed to be benign.[7–9] Features that warrant further evaluation and a higher suspicion for an STS are a size greater than 5 cm, the mass is deep to the muscle fascia and a history of rapid growth.[10]

Most patients with STS present with a painless mass and only rarely exhibit constitutional cancer symptoms such as weight loss and malaise.[11] As such, the clinician should approach all soft-tissue masses with a high index of suspicion and obtain a detailed history and physical.

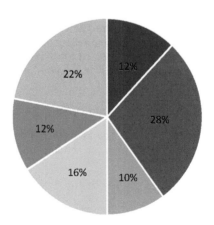

■ Upper extremity   ■ Lower extremity   ■ Trunk   ■ Retroperitoneal   ■ Other   ■ Visceral

Fig. 1. Locations of soft-tissue sarcomas.[4]

EPIDEMIOLOGY

Many patients with STS are younger adults, but it can occur at any age and with equal gender distribution.[11,12]Although most STSs are sporadic in etiology, risk factors include exposure to ionizing radiation or chemicals such as herbicides/pesticides (phenoxy acetic acid, dioxin, and chlorophenols).[3,11,13] Patients who undergo unplanned excisions tend to present with earlier stage disease, as seen in a study by *Alamanda and colleagues*[14]where 63.7% of those with unplanned excisions had American Joint Committee on Cancer (AJCC) stages I and II disease compared with only 39.7% of those who underwent primary oncologic excision ($P < .05$). This study also showed that patients with smaller (median size of 5 cm) vs larger tumors (median size of 12 cm) were more likely to have unplanned excisions ($P < .05$), especially if the tumor site was in the upper extremity.[14] Although some reports have conflicting findings, it is generally accepted that superficial tumors have a higher association with unplanned excisions vs deeper, fixed masses.[15]

DIAGNOSTIC WORKUP

Unplanned excisions are classified into two categories: total unplanned excision and partial unplanned excision.[11] It was Giuliano and Eilber,[16] and subsequently, *Noria and colleagues*,[17] who first used the term "total unplanned excision" to refer to tumor resection without any preoperative diagnostic studies or an intent to obtain cancer-free margins.[11] This type of excision usually is seen in nonspecialized centers and among patients who present with smaller and more superficial soft-tissue masses.[11] Partial unplanned excisions occur less frequently, only in about 11% to 34% of patients.[11,15,18] These excisions have some degree of preoperative planning via imaging and/or biopsy performed, but the results are frequently insufficient or misinterpreted, leading to a non-oncologic excision.[11,15,18]

According to guidelines, MRI is the gold-standard imaging for an extremity or truncal mass suspicious for an STS, as it can determine the depth and the anatomic relationship to nearby muscles and critical neurovascular bundles.[12,19] Before obtaining an MRI, ultrasound could be used to initially assess for suspicious tumor characteristics such as irregular shape, depth, and increased vascularity.[20] However, this is primarily useful for smaller, superficial lesions that otherwise seem benign as it is a low cost and a readily available modality to determine if further workup is needed.[20] A CT can also be helpful, but it is more commonly used for abdominal or retroperitoneal lesions or for chest staging in high-grade tumors to assess for pulmonary metastases.[12,21]

If there is suspicion of STS based on examination and imaging, a core needle biopsy is the preferred mode of tissue sampling to obtain a diagnosis due to its accuracy and low risk for complications.[22] Histologically, the diagnosis of STS is made based on morphologic patterns and immunohistochemical staining. Translocation or amplification of certain genes has been noted among various histologic subtypes, including the amplification of MDM2 and CDK4 in liposarcomas.[23] If a larger amount of tissue is needed for flow cytometry or the analysis of chromosomal translocations, incisional biopsy is appropriate. However, this must be carefully planned to account for future surgical resection and cosmetic reconstruction (**Box 1**).[11,24,25]As such, it is generally recommended that an incisional biopsy is performed by a surgeon who will be performing the oncologic resection, as this can ensure that the biopsy site is placed longitudinally along the extremity, so the scar may be resected en bloc at the time of definitive surgery to prevent tumor cell dissemination.[24,25]

Box 1
Principles for biopsy in soft-tissue sarcoma[11]

1. Perform the biopsy over the tumor and in line with the planned definitive surgical incision.

2. Only violate one compartment of tissue so as not to contaminate adjacent vessels, nerves, or joints.

3. Obtain meticulous hemostasis to avoid hematoma formation and subsequent contamination or distortion of planes.

4. If drains are placed, place them close to and in line with the planned definitive surgical incision.

MANAGEMENT CONSIDERATIONS

Unplanned excisions will almost never result in the oncologically appropriate negative margins achieved by an appropriately planned surgical wide resection for a known STS. Consequently, 24% to 91% of patients with unplanned excisions have a gross or microscopic residual tumor.[6,8,11,13,16,17,26] Guidelines recommend that en bloc STS removal should occur through normal uninvolved tissue outside of any tumor pseudocapsule with at least 1 cm margins or inclusion of a fascial barrier.[12] This is to fully encompass local tumor spread and thus decrease the rate of locoregional recurrence.[7] STS surgical management also prioritizes the preservation of function, particularly in extremity lesions. In the unplanned excision scenario, neoadjuvant therapy with radiation, chemotherapy, or both is no longer available as part of the multimodality treatment of STS. The use of these treatments is often based on size, location, histologic subtype, and grade of the STS and best incorporated under the guidance of a multidisciplinary group of experts before any initial surgical excision (**Fig. 2**).

The overall impact of non-oncologic, unplanned excisions on the outcome of patients with extremity STS is complex. There are various factors to be considered when presented with a patient who has undergone a non-oncologic resection. These include the location of the tumor, presence of positive margins (macroscopic vs

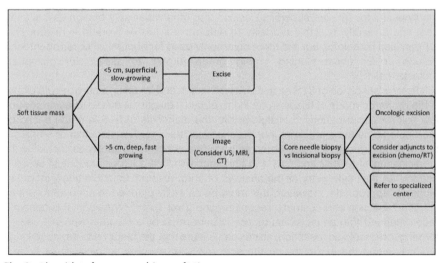

Fig. 2. Algorithm for approaching soft-tissue masses.

microscopic), the prior surgical incision, presence of a hematoma or surgical drains, and the grade and size of the tumor.[11] Consequently, all patients with an STS diagnosis should be referred to a high-volume specialty center as this is associated with improved short-term and long-term patient outcomes.[27]

As compared with planned oncologic wide resection, unplanned excisions of STS have consistently been associated with worse 5-year local recurrence-free survival (RFS).[6–8,11,13,17] In a study by *Potter and colleagues*, 5-year RFS was only 63.7% after unplanned excisions vs 89.7% for planned resection ($P < .0001$).[13] This study also noted that, after excision of the tumor bed, the residual microscopic disease was associated with decreased disease-specific survival compared with no residual disease (69.8% vs 87.5%; $P = .06$).[13] Other studies, such as *Chandrasekar and colleagues*,[8] have shown similar findings with a recurrence risk ratio of 3.07 noted for patients, with residual tumor after re-resection ($P = .0037$). As such, complete resection of STS—is it initially or with a salvage resection—remains crucial to the local management.

Although many studies that have shown worse locoregional RFS in patients who underwent unplanned resection attribute the poorer outcomes to an inadequate initial resection that contaminated the surgical field with malignant cells, some studies suggest that referral to a specialty center with salvage wide resection can still result in overall acceptable oncologic outcomes.[9,26,28] In a propensity-matched, multi-institutional study comparing the outcomes of unplanned STS excisions vs planned resections, locoregional RFS was worse for unplanned excision patients with high-grade STS, but there was no statistically significant difference between the groups in terms of distant metastasis-free survival and disease-specific survival.[7] Consequently, although STS patients who undergo unplanned excision have a higher risk for local recurrence, particularly with high-grade tumors, there does not seem to be an associated decrease in overall survival (OS).

Although there are over 100 histologic STS subtypes, the most common extremity subtypes include liposarcoma, leiomyosarcoma, and undifferentiated pleomorphic sarcoma (UPS).[1] The specific histology will have some impact on both local recurrence and OS. Liposarcomas arise from the same cells that form adipocytes and are further subclassified as well differentiated, dedifferentiated, myxoid/round cell, or pleomorphic—all of which have differences in local recurrence and survival outcomes.[29] Well-differentiated liposarcomas, for example, have a very favorable prognosis. These tumors can be excised without wide margins due to their low rate of local recurrence, and they are almost never treated with preoperative or postoperative radiation.[1] Dedifferentiated liposarcomas, on the other hand, are the high-grade counterparts of well differentiated liposarcoma. The 5-year OS rate for dedifferentiated liposarcoma is approximately 45%, and radiation is frequently used to reduce the risk for local recurrence.[29] Myxoid liposarcomas are the most radiosensitive of the liposarcoma subtypes. Although their risk for local recurrence is low, they do have a greater tendency to metastasize to extrapulmonary sites; therefore, chemotherapy is sometimes considered in their management.[30] Pleomorphic liposarcomas are very aggressive, frequently demonstrating high rates of both local recurrence and early distant metastases.[31]

Leiomyosarcomas have an overall lower risk for local recurrence (~6%) but a higher rate of distant metastases (~46%).[32] This histologic subtype tends to have a preference for the lower limb, and preoperative or postoperative radiation is often considered for tumors greater than 5 cm in size, especially high grade.[1,33]

Unlike leiomyosarcomas, which have limited sensitivity to chemotherapy, UPS has been identified as a more chemo-responsive STS subtype in multiple studies.[7,34] These tumors have intermediate outcomes with local recurrence and distant metastatic rates of 30% to 35%.[35]

THERAPEUTIC OPTIONS FOR THE UNPLANNED EXCISION
Salvage Wide Resection

Unless the associated morbidity is prohibitive, formal salvage wide resection of the unplanned STS excision site should be considered as the potentially curative treatment.[6,13] Wide resection should include en bloc removal of the entire prior operative site, including the surgical scar and drain tracts, as well as oncologically appropriate margins of adjacent uninvolved soft tissue to fully encompass the prior STS location.[11] Salvage wide resection tends to be more complicated than what would have been oncologically appropriate for the STS at initial presentation before the unplanned excision and is thus associated with increased surgical and functional morbidity.[8,11,13]Because of the contamination of adjacent, previously uninvolved tissues from the use of transverse incisions, drains placed outside of the line of resection, postoperative hematomas that violate tissue planes, and spillage of a gross tumor, multiple studies have shown a more frequent need for resections requiring complex plastic surgery reconstruction and consideration for radiation therapy in addition to surgery.[7,11,36] In addition, ill-defined scar tissue, the lack of a palpable mass for guidance, and loss of normal anatomic planes also complicates the technical aspects of salvage wide resection.[11]

Despite the potential associated morbidity, salvage wide resection has shown to be an independent predictor of improved local control. In a study by *Morii and colleagues*[37] comparing patients who underwent salvage wide resection vs nonoperative management of STS with radiation or chemotherapy, 5-year local RFS was superior for surgery (87.9% vs 49.9%; $P = .002$).

Radiation

Radiation therapy is an adjunct to STS surgical wide resection and can be administered either preoperatively or postoperatively. The National Comprehensive Cancer Network recommends radiation for stage II or higher tumors, although surgery alone can be considered sufficient for stage I tumors that undergo wide resection.[38] For planned wide resection, preoperative radiation is often considered to optimize dosing to the tumor, sterilize margins along with critical structures, and increase the chance of limb preservation, particularly for large-grade or high-grade STS.[1] Although the role of radiation has been well established through multiple clinical trials, particularly in extremity STS,[39,40] the optimal sequencing of radiation with surgery (preoperative vs postoperative) is a complex and nuanced decision.[1]

The role of radiation in the unplanned sarcoma excision is still not well defined.[13,41,42] In a retrospective study of patients who underwent unplanned STS excisions treated only with postoperative radiation (no salvage wide resection), local control at 10-year was 86%.[41] However, several other studies have shown that radiation alone is not effective in preventing local recurrence after unplanned excisions.[11,13,42,43]As such, combining radiation with salvage wide resection to maximize local control for unplanned STS excisions at very high risk for local recurrence can be considered. A study by *Jones and colleagues*[44] demonstrated an 86% 5-year RFS for unplanned STS excision patients treated with preoperative radiation followed by salvage wide resection.

Chemotherapy

The role of chemotherapy in the treatment of STS is typically limited to patients at very high risk for developing or already having distant metastatic disease. In a phase 3 randomized trial of patients with greater than 5 cm, deep, and high-grade truncal and extremity STS treated with neoadjuvant chemotherapy (anthracycline and ifosfamide), chemotherapy was associated with a 62% disease-free survival at approximately 4-year period.[45] Other smaller studies have suggested that there may be a high-risk cohort of STS patients—particularly those with high-grade tumors that are greater than 10 cm—who may benefit from neoadjuvan tchemotherapy.[46,47] Moreover, combining preoperative radiation with chemotherapy has also shown to be feasible.[48] When the primary STS is still present, one of the potential benefits of neoadjuvant chemotherapy is that the primary tumor can act as an "in vivo" marker of any potential treatment response. If the primary tumor did not respond to chemotherapy after a few initial cycles, then chemotherapy would be discontinued. This theoretic benefit is lost in the setting of a previously unplanned excision.

Adjuvant chemotherapy can also be considered following the definitive treatment of the primary STS site. A meta-analysis of 18 chemotherapy trials showed only a marginal OS benefit to adjuvant chemotherapy compared with surgery alone among patients with localized, resectable STS (Hazard Ratio (HR) 0.77; $P = .01$).[49]Interestingly, one study has shown that the 5-year survival of STS patients receiving chemotherapy after unplanned excision was lower than patients who did not receive chemotherapy.[15] Consequently, the role of chemotherapy in the treatment of an STS patient with an unplanned excision should be determined on a case-by-case basis based on the calculated risk of developing distant metastatic disease and any anticipated potential improvement in survival.

SUMMARY

In summary, STS is a rare disease with variable outcomes that should be managed at specialized sarcoma centers where there is a multidisciplinary expert team. Unplanned excisions occur in up to 50% of patients with STS and are associated with increased local recurrence due to possible seeding of the tumor bed with malignant cells. Thus, salvage wide resection is generally recommended following unplanned excision but can be associated with increased morbidity, the need for reconstructive surgery, or even amputation. Disease recurrence and survival vary based on multiple STS factors, including histologic subtypes. Radiation and/or chemotherapy are adjuncts that can be considered in addition to resection to improve outcomes. Considering STS on the differential of possibilities for a soft-tissue mass, appropriate preoperative three-dimensional imaging, and strong consideration for core needle biopsy to make a definitive pathologic diagnosis are all factors that can reduce the likelihood of an unplanned STS excision.

CLINICS CARE POINTS

- A high index of suspicion, preoperative imaging, and core needle biopsy can reduce the possibility of misinterpreting soft-tissue sarcoma (STS) as a benign mass.

- Unplanned excisions of STS have been associated with decreased local recurrence-free survival.

- Salvage wide resection should be considered for an unplanned STS excision if the associated morbidity is acceptable.

- Management of STS at high-volume, specialized centers is associated with improved oncologic outcomes.

DISCLOSURE

The authors have nothing to disclose.

REFERENCES

1. Gamboa AC, Gronchi A, Cardona K. Soft-tissue sarcoma in adults: An update on the current state of histiotype-specific management in an era of personalized medicine. CaCancer J Clin 2020;70(3):200–29.
2. Blay JY, Honoré C, Stoeckle E, et al. Surgery in reference centers improves survival of sarcoma patients: a nationwide study. Ann Oncol 2019;30(7):1143–53.
3. Siegel HJ, Brown O, Lopez-Ben R, et al. Unplanned surgical excision of extremity soft tissue sarcomas: patient profile and referral patterns. J SurgOrthop Adv 2009;18(2):93–8.
4. Brennan MF, Antonescu CR, Moraco N, et al. Lessons learned from the study of 10,000 patients with soft tissue sarcoma. Ann Surg 2014;260(3):416–21 [discussion: 421-412].
5. Lawrence W, Donegan WL, Natarajan N, et al. Adult soft tissue sarcomas. A pattern of care survey of the American College of Surgeons. Ann Surg 1987; 205(4):349–59.
6. Lewis JJ, Leung D, Espat J, et al. Effect of reresection in extremity soft tissue sarcoma. Ann Surg 2000;231(5):655–63.
7. Zaidi MY, Ethun CG, Liu Y, et al. The impact of unplanned excisions of truncal/extremity soft tissue sarcomas: A multi-institutional propensity score analysis from the US Sarcoma Collaborative. J SurgOncol 2019;120(3):332–9.
8. Chandrasekar CR, Wafa H, Grimer RJ, et al. The effect of an unplanned excision of a soft-tissue sarcoma on prognosis. JBoneJointSurg Br 2008;90(2):203–8.
9. Smolle MA, Tunn PU, Goldenitsch E, et al. The prognostic impact of unplanned excisions in a cohort of 728 soft tissue sarcoma patients: a multicentre study. Ann SurgOncol 2017;24(6):1596–605.
10. Hussein R, Smith MA. Soft tissue sarcomas: are current referral guidelines sufficient? Ann R CollSurg Engl 2005;87(3):171–3.
11. Pretell-Mazzini J, Barton MD, Conway SA, et al. Unplanned excision of soft-tissue sarcomas: current concepts for management and prognosis. JBoneJointSurg Am 2015;97(7):597–603.
12. Cameron JL, Cameron AM. Current surgical therapy. Philadelphia, PA: Elsevier; 2017.
13. Potter BK, Adams SC, Pitcher JD, et al. Local recurrence of disease after unplanned excisions of high-grade soft tissue sarcomas. ClinOrthopRelat Res 2008;466(12):3093–100.
14. Alamanda VK, Delisca GO, Archer KR, et al. Incomplete excisions of extremity soft tissue sarcomas are unaffected by insurance status or distance from a sarcoma center. J SurgOncol 2013;108(7):477–80.
15. Hoshi M, Ieguchi M, Takami M, et al. Clinical problems after initial unplanned resection of sarcoma. Jpn J ClinOncol 2008;38(10):701–9.
16. Giuliano AE, Eilber FR. The rationale for planned reoperation after unplanned total excision of soft-tissue sarcomas. J ClinOncol 1985;3(10):1344–8.
17. Noria S, Davis A, Kandel R, et al. Residual disease following unplanned excision of soft-tissue sarcoma of an extremity. J BoneJointSurg Am 1996;78(5):650–5.
18. Davies AM, Mehr A, Parsonage S, et al. MR imaging in the assessment of residual tumour following inadequate primary excision of soft tissue sarcomas. EurRadiol 2004;14(3):506–13.
19. Sundaram M, McGuire MH, Herbold DR. Magnetic resonance imaging of soft tissue masses: an evaluation of fifty-three histologically proven tumors. MagnResonImaging 1988;6(3):237–48.

20. Hung EH, Griffith JF. Pitfalls in ultrasonography of soft tissue tumors. SeminMusculoskeletRadiol 2014;18(1):79–85.
21. Mohammed TL, Chowdhry A, Reddy GP, et al. ACR Appropriateness Criteria® screening for pulmonary metastases. J ThoracImaging 2011;26(1):W1–3.
22. Strauss DC, Qureshi YA, Hayes AJ, et al. The role of core needle biopsy in the diagnosis of suspected soft tissue tumours. J SurgOncol 2010;102(5):523–9.
23. Conyers R, Young S, Thomas DM. Liposarcoma: molecular genetics and therapeutics. Sarcoma 2011;2011:483154.
24. Mankin HJ, Lange TA, Spanier SS. The hazards of biopsy in patients with malignant primary bone and soft-tissue tumors. J BoneJointSurg Am 1982;64(8): 1121–7.
25. Mankin HJ, Mankin CJ, Simon MA. The hazards of the biopsy, revisited. Members of the Musculoskeletal Tumor Society. J BoneJointSurg Am 1996;78(5):656–63.
26. Fiore M, Casali PG, Miceli R, et al. Prognostic effect of re-excision in adult soft tissue sarcoma of the extremity. Ann SurgOncol 2006;13(1):110–7.
27. Begg CB, Cramer LD, Hoskins WJ, et al. Impact of hospital volume on operative mortality for major cancer surgery. JAMA 1998;280(20):1747–51.
28. Bianchi G, Sambri A, Cammelli S, et al. Impact of residual disease after "unplanned excision" of primary localized adult soft tissue sarcoma of the extremities: evaluation of 452 cases at a single Institution. Musculoskelet Surg 2017; 101(3):243–8.
29. Vos M, Koseła-Paterczyk H, Rutkowski P, et al. Differences in recurrence and survival of extremity liposarcoma subtypes. Eur J SurgOncol 2018;44(9):1391–7.
30. Schwab JH, Boland P, Guo T, et al. Skeletal metastases in myxoidliposarcoma: an unusual pattern of distant spread. Ann SurgOncol 2007;14(4):1507–14.
31. Oliveira AM, Nascimento AG. Pleomorphic liposarcoma. SeminDiagnPathol 2001; 18(4):274–85.
32. Abraham JA, Weaver MJ, Hornick JL, et al. Outcomes and prognostic factors for a consecutive case series of 115 patients with somatic leiomyosarcoma. J BoneJointSurg Am 2012;94(8):736–44.
33. Massi D, Beltrami G, Mela MM, et al. Prognostic factors in soft tissue leiomyosarcoma of the extremities: a retrospective analysis of 42 cases. Eur J SurgOncol 2004;30(5):565–72.
34. Stacchiotti S, Verderio P, Messina A, et al. Tumor response assessment by modified Choi criteria in localized high-risk soft tissue sarcoma treated with chemotherapy. Cancer 2012;118(23):5857–66.
35. Widemann BC, Italiano A. Biology and Management of Undifferentiated Pleomorphic Sarcoma, Myxofibrosarcoma, and Malignant Peripheral Nerve Sheath Tumors: State of the Art and Perspectives. J ClinOncol 2018;36(2):160–7.
36. Sugiura H, Takahashi M, Katagiri H, et al. Additional wide resection of malignant soft tissue tumors. ClinOrthopRelat Res 2002;394:201–10.
37. Morii T, Yabe H, Morioka H, et al. Clinical significance of additional wide resection for unplanned resection of high grade soft tissue sarcoma. OpenOrthop J 2008;2: 126–9.
38. Network NCC. Soft tissue sarcoma.Version 2.2021. National Comprehensive Cancer Network; 2021.
39. Pisters PW, Harrison LB, Leung DH, et al. Long-term results of a prospective randomized trial of adjuvant brachytherapy in soft tissue sarcoma. J ClinOncol 1996; 14(3):859–68.

40. Yang JC, Chang AE, Baker AR, et al. Randomized prospective study of the benefit of adjuvant radiation therapy in the treatment of soft tissue sarcomas of the extremity. J ClinOncol 1998;16(1):197–203.
41. Kepka L, Suit HD, Goldberg SI, et al. Results of radiation therapy performed after unplanned surgery (without re-excision) for soft tissue sarcomas. J SurgOncol 2005;92(1):39–45.
42. Manoso MW, Pratt J, Healey JH, et al. Infiltrative MRI pattern and incomplete initial surgery compromise local control of myxofibrosarcoma. ClinOrthopRelat Res 2006;450:89–94.
43. Lin PP, Guzel VB, Pisters PW, et al. Surgical management of soft tissue sarcomas of the hand and foot. Cancer 2002;95(4):852–61.
44. Jones DA, Shideman C, Yuan J, et al. Management of Unplanned Excision for Soft-Tissue Sarcoma With Preoperative Radiotherapy Followed by Definitive Resection. Am J ClinOncol 2016;39(6):586–92.
45. Gronchi A, Ferrari S, Quagliuolo V, et al. Histotype-tailored neoadjuvant chemotherapy versus standard chemotherapy in patients with high-risk soft-tissue sarcomas (ISG-STS 1001): an international, open-label, randomised, controlled, phase 3, multicentre trial. LancetOncol 2017;18(6):812–22.
46. Meric F, Hess KR, Varma DG, et al. Radiographic response to neoadjuvant chemotherapy is a predictor of local control and survival in soft tissue sarcomas. Cancer 2002;95(5):1120–6.
47. Grobmyer SR, Maki RG, Demetri GD, et al. Neo-adjuvant chemotherapy for primary high-grade extremity soft tissue sarcoma. Ann Oncol 2004;15(11):1667–72.
48. Palassini E, Ferrari S, Verderio P, et al. Feasibility of Preoperative Chemotherapy With or Without Radiation Therapy in Localized Soft Tissue Sarcomas of Limbs and Superficial Trunk in the Italian Sarcoma Group/GrupoEspañol de Investigación en Sarcomas Randomized Clinical Trial: Three Versus Five Cycles of Full-Dose Epirubicin Plus Ifosfamide. J ClinOncol 2015;33(31):3628–34.
49. Pervaiz N, Colterjohn N, Farrokhyar F, et al. A systematic meta-analysis of randomized controlled trials of adjuvant chemotherapy for localized resectable soft-tissue sarcoma. Cancer 2008;113(3):573–81.

The Role of Imaging in Soft Tissue Sarcoma Diagnosis and Management

Cimarron E. Sharon, MD, Richard J. Straker III, MD,
Giorgos C. Karakousis, MD*

KEYWORDS

- Soft tissue sarcomas • Computed tomography • Magnetic resonance imaging
- ^{18}F-FDG PET-CT • Ultrasound

KEY POINTS

- Ultrasound (US) and magnetic resonance imaging (MRI) are useful initial radiologic diagnostic modalities for the assessment and characterization of a soft tissue mass.
- Staging of soft tissue sarcomas (STSs) should include chest imaging, ideally in the form of a computed tomography (CT) of the chest. Imaging of the abdomen/pelvis is generally limited to specific histologic subtypes of sarcoma with a propensity to extrathoracic metastasis.
- Soft tissue masses, particularly those >3cm, with any radiographic concern for malignancy should generally be biopsied before surgical resection, ideally guided by US or CT to target the most representative cellular (non-necrotic) portion of the lesion.
- Postsurgical surveillance of the primary tumor site with US or MRI should be performed every 3 to 6 months with surveillance chest imaging accordingly.
- ^{18}F-fluorodeoxyglucose positron emission tomography-CT generally plays a more limited role in STS management but may be helpful in assessing response to therapy for certain subtypes.

INTRODUCTION

The differential diagnosis of a soft tissue mass is broad, and an appropriate imaging workup is crucial to accurate identification. Additionally, imaging plays a critical role in soft tissue sarcoma (STS) staging and monitoring for disease progression. In this article, we discuss the different imaging modalities and their utility in the workup and surveillance of STS.

Department of Surgery, Hospital of the University of Pennsylvania, 3400 Spruce Street, Philadelphia, PA 19104, USA
* Corresponding author.
E-mail address: giorgos.karakousis@uphs.upenn.edu

Surg Clin N Am 102 (2022) 539–550
https://doi.org/10.1016/j.suc.2022.04.003   surgical.theclinics.com
0039-6109/22/© 2022 Elsevier Inc. All rights reserved.

INITIAL DIAGNOSTIC IMAGING
Plain Radiographs

Plain radiographs may be a valuable first step in the evaluation of a soft tissue mass. Radiographs are widely available, low cost, afford minimal radiation exposure to the patient,[1] and can provide useful diagnostic information for STSs.[2,3] Additionally, radiographs can identify bone density lesions (ie, myositis ossifications and osteochondroma)[4] that can present as a palpable mass, which would alter the subsequent diagnostic evaluation. For STS specifically, radiographs identify calcification and ossification, of which certain patterns point to specific pathologic diagnoses. For example, synovial sarcomas tend to have coarse, amorphous, or spiculated calcifications,[5,6] hemangiomas can contain multiple punctate round lesions described as pleboliths,[7] and liposarcomas might have large and coarse calcifications.[4] Plain radiographs may also assist in identifying bone involvement by an STS although this finding is more readily visualized with computed tomography (CT) and magnetic resonance imaging (MRI), which are discussed later in this article. Although often easily obtainable and low cost, plain radiographs are generally inadequate for planning the surgical resection of soft tissue masses, where cross-sectional imaging is desirable for better delineation of anatomic considerations.

Ultrasound

Ultrasound (US), much like plain radiographs, is an easily accessible and affordable imaging modality frequently used in the initial assessment of a soft tissue mass, which has the added benefit of not exposing the patient to any radiation.[8] Specific strengths of US include distinguishing between a benign cyst versus a cystic appearing mass, and assessing the vascularity of a lesion, which is performed through the addition of color Doppler.[9] The presence of internal vascularity identified on Doppler is considered a concerning imaging finding, which would typically prompt further diagnostic workup.[10] Additional findings consistent with an STS include a hemorrhagic component[11] and a heterogeneous appearance.[10] Additionally, a tumor size greater than 3 cm is considered a worrisome finding.[12] US also affords the ability to diagnose certain benign soft tissue masses which have characteristic sonographic appearances (eg, lipomas, peripheral nerve sheath tumors), thus potentially obviating the need for further workup. If any concerning features are identified on US, then further imaging with MRI is typically recommended. It is worth noting that the utility of US is generally limited to tumors that are superficial as it its ability to provide high resolution for deeper-seated lesions is limited. Additionally, US is operator dependent and may not be applicable in centers with limited experience in soft tissue US. **Fig. 1** demonstrates an US of a patient with a liposarcoma of the calf.

Magnetic Resonance Imaging

MRI is generally considered the optimal imaging modality for the evaluation of soft tissue lesions of the trunk and extremity[8,13] and is preferred by the American College of Radiology.[14] MRI's excellent tissue contrast and multiplanar imaging provides superior information regarding the tumor's relationship to adjacent structures, including the vasculature, bone, nerves, and muscle.[13,15-18] In some instances, MRI can point the diagnosis toward specific subtypes of sarcoma [ie well-differentiated liposarcoma (WDLPS)], based on classic imaging findings. If MRI is not available, then CT can provide helpful diagnostic and anatomic information although it is not the preferred imaging modality for initial workup of a soft tissue mass of the head and neck, trunk, or extremity. In contrast, CT is preferred in the evaluation of retroperitoneal sarcomas.[19]

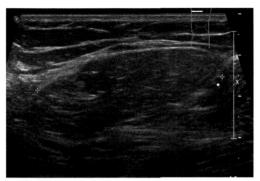

Fig. 1. Ultrasound findings of a 48-year-old man with an R calf mass. Ultrasound showed a well-encapsulated mass similar in echotexture to the surrounding fat, which measured 1.8 × 4.6 × 5.7 cm without vascularity identified on Doppler. This was biopsied due to the size and was found to be a liposarcoma.

MRI includes a combination of T1, T2, and diffusion-weighted images (DWIs), which help delineate tumor anatomy and, in some cases, even the pathologic diagnosis. In T1-weighted images, adipose tissue is hyperintense, whereas on T2-weighted images fluid is hyperintense. On DWI, the degree of brightness on imaging correlates to the rate of water diffusion. The combination of findings seen on all these MRI modalities assists in the characterization of tumor anatomy and malignancy.[20,21] Areas with low T1 and high T2 intensity are indicative of free water and help distinguish tumor edge from surrounding edema.[22] Gadolinium contrast administration during MRI identifies the degree of tumor vascularity and invasion of surrounding vessels.[22] Additionally, the areas of the tumor with the most contrast enhancement correspond to the pathologic regions with the highest grade.[23]

MRI findings can help narrow the differential diagnosis of an STS. Overall, T1 signal heterogeneity and the absence of a low T2 signal have a high sensitivity in diagnosing a malignant lesion.[24] However, the specific diagnosis can be further elucidated based on classical imaging characteristics. Lesions with high T1 and low T2 intensity represent fat and are commonly indicative of lipomatous tumors; WDLPS consists mostly of fat but can demonstrate thick septations, associated nonlipomatous masses, foci of high T2 signal, and areas of enhancement.[25] Sarcomas with a high T1- and T2-weighted signal typically represent clear cell sarcomas or sarcomas with a hemorrhagic component.[3] The vast majority of sarcomas demonstrate an intermediate T1 signal and high T2 intensity.[26] **Fig. 2** demonstrates MRI findings of a patient with an atypical lipomatous tumor of the thigh.

Computed Tomography

If MRI is contraindicated, then CT with intravenous contrast is the diagnostic imaging modality of choice for the initial evaluation of a soft tissue mass.[27] In general, MRI is preferred to CT as CT results in more radiation exposure and less contrast resolution. Additionally, CT scans frequently overestimate the size of the tumor, as CT does not reliably distinguish between the tumor itself and the surrounding edema.[28] However, CT angiography can provide valuable information regarding tumor vascularity, vascular involvement and can help distinguish cystic from solid tumors.[29,30]

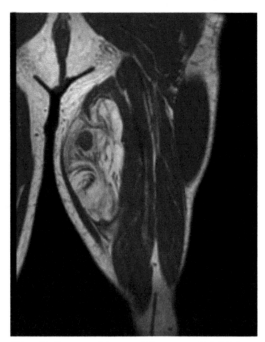

Fig. 2. T1-weighted MRI of a 53-year-old man with an L medial thigh mass. Imaging demonstrates a large region of hyperintensity consistent with adipose tissue, with a discrete hypointense region consistent with focal de-differentiation. Pathology was consistent with an atypical lipomatous tumor.

^{18}F-Fluorodeoxyglucose Positron Emission Tomography-Computed Tomography

According to the American College of Radiology's appropriateness guidelines, ^{18}F-FDG PET-CT is not recommended for the initial workup of an STS.[27] However, it is worth noting that uptake by ^{18}F-FDG, a glucose analog, is directly correlated with histologic grade, mitotic activity, and p53 expression.[31,32] Additionally, a higher standardized uptake value (SUV), indicating higher glucose utilization and cellular activity, has been shown to correlate with a shorter disease-free interval and worse overall survival.[33,34] The utility of ^{18}F-FDG PET-CT in staging and disease surveillance will be discussed later in this article.

IMAGE-GUIDED BIOPSY

Following appropriate imaging workup, obtaining a tissue diagnosis is crucial for developing a treatment plan. Core needle biopsy is most frequently used, due to its low complication profile and high diagnostic accuracy.[35,36] US and CT can be used to assist in obtaining a biopsy; the choice of modality is dependent on the radiologist's preference and the anatomic site and location of the highest grade tumor component.[4] It is critical to obtain imaging before tissue biopsy, as prebiopsy imaging identifies the areas of the tumor with potentially the highest pathologic grade, which should be targeted during biopsy. Additionally, postbiopsy hemorrhage and edema can alter the appearance of the tumor on imaging,[37] which could cause diagnostic confusion if no prebiopsy images were obtained.

STAGING
Chest Imaging

Due to the propensity of STS for hematogenous metastasis to the lungs, dedicated chest imaging is critical for the appropriate staging of patients. The American Joint Committee on Cancer (AJCC) 8th edition,[38] as well as the European Society for Medical Oncology (ESMO) guidelines,[39] recommends a chest CT to assess for pulmonary metastases in patients with STS. However, the American College of Radiology[40] and the National Comprehensive Center Network (NCCN) guidelines[41] state that either a chest CT or chest X-ray (CXR) is acceptable for this purpose. A chest CT affords the opportunity to identify subcentimeter lung nodules earlier and assess for any interval growth, which may impact care of the patient before the identification of the lesions by CXR.

Abdominal/Pelvic Imaging

It is very uncommon for most STS to metastasize to lymph nodes, and generally, lymphadenectomy is not part of the surgical management. However, the presence of lymph node metastases, although still relatively uncommon, has been described in specific histologic subtypes, such as angiosarcoma, epithelioid sarcoma, and clear cell sarcoma.[42–45] Additionally, round cell and myxoid liposarcoma can present with extrapulmonary metastases, specifically to abdominal and retroperitoneal viscera.[46,47] As such, for these specific subtypes, a dedicated CT of the abdomen and pelvis should be considered to assess for lymph node and/or abdominal metastases.[48]

18F-Fluorodeoxyglucose Positron Emission Tomography-Computed Tomography

The role of [18]FDG-PET-CT in staging is generally limited in the management of STS. It has the ability to identify increased metabolic activity in normal-sized lymph nodes, which may be missed by CT alone,[49] and may play a limited role in the initial staging of certain subtypes (eg, myxoid/round cell) with potential intra-abdominal metastases. However, as previously discussed, lymph node metastases are exceedingly uncommon and are unique to only a few histologic subtypes. In regard to detection of pulmonary metastases, [18]FDG-PET-CT has been shown to be less sensitive[50–52] but more specific than a chest CT.[50,51] In one institutional study of 75 patients with STS, only one patient was upstaged based on [18]FDG-PET-CT findings compared with CT alone.[52] [18]FDG-PET-CT is thus unlikely to alter management in STS patients, and given the cost and radiation exposure, it is not typically recommended. The main utility of [18]FDG-PET-CT for STS is in monitoring response to therapy.

Rare Sites of Metastases

Clear cell sarcomas, alveolar soft part sarcomas, and angiosarcomas have a tendency to metastasize to the brain.[53–55] As such, both ESMO and NCCN guidelines recommend a dedicated CT or MRI of the brain for patients with extremity STS and these pathologies.[39,56] Additionally, myxoid and round cell liposarcoma have a high risk of metastases to the spine, and as such, an MRI of the total spine should be considered as part of the staging evaluation.[57–59]

SURGICAL PLANNING

It is critical for a surgeon to carefully review preoperative imaging to assess tumor resectability. Initial staging imaging can help guide indications for surgery (ie, whether palliative or curative in intent). Diagnostic imaging of the primary tumor site will identify

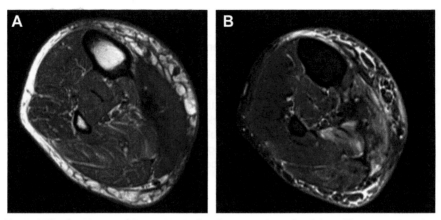

Fig. 3. MRI of a 48-year-old man 2 months after resection of a right calf sarcoma. Imaging shows edema of the surgical bed, which is hyperintense on T1 (*A*) and hypointense on short tau inversion recovery (STIR) (*B*), a fat suppression technique.

any important anatomic considerations for resection (eg, neurovascular or bony involvement), allowing for counseling of patients with respect to any anticipated functional sequalae from surgery. Preoperative imaging should be carefully reviewed by a multidisciplinary team to also make decisions about the sequencing of treatment, including radiation and systemic therapies.

SURVEILLANCE

Due to the heterogeneity of STS, it is challenging to identify literature on effective surveillance strategies[60–62] Typically, recommendations vary by tumor pathology and stage. Regardless of the time interval chosen for assessment, it is imperative to compare all surveillance images to those performed pretreatment as tumor recurrence traditionally appears as a discrete region with similar imaging characteristics of the original tumor.[4]

Postsurgical Surveillance

Following surgical resection, per NCCN guidelines, it is recommended that patients undergo a history and physical (H&P) every 3 to 6 months for up to 3 years, and then annually.[48] Chest imaging should be obtained every 6 to 12 months, and a chest CT is preferred to plain radiographs.[48] Imaging of the primary site should occur based on the individualized risk of local recurrence, typically every 3 to 6 months. Imaging modalities to assess local recurrence include US and MRI for extremity and truncal lesions, depending on the depth of the original tumor. CT abdomen and pelvis are generally performed for retroperitoneal sarcomas although MRI can also be considered for this anatomic location. One retrospective study found no significant difference between US and MRI for detecting local recurrence.[63] Another showed that US has a high sensitivity and specificity (92% and 94%, respectively).[64] However, as previously discussed, US is operator dependent and requires institutional expertise in the surveillance of soft tissue tumors. Additionally, in the early postoperative period, there can be more challenges to the interpretation of US findings in terms of distinguishing expected postoperative changes from recurrent or residual disease.[63] In contrast, MRI can more reliably distinguish tumor from postoperative hemorrhage or seroma.

Fig. 3 demonstrates a postoperative MRI of a patient who underwent resection of a calf liposarcoma.

In one study of patients with mostly undifferentiated pleomorphic sarcoma, [18]FDG-PET-CT demonstrated similar sensitivity and specificity to MRI in detecting tumor recurrence.[65] However, [18]FDG-PET-CT is generally not used despite it having the potential advantage of simultaneously detecting local and distant recurrences.[4] In the early postoperative period, PET/CT can also be limited by the inability to distinguish residual/recurrent disease from expected postoperative changes. In some cases, [18]FDG-PET-CT could be considered if MRI is contraindicated.

Monitoring Response to Therapy

The Response Evaluation Criteria in Solid Tumors (RECIST) is the current method used to assess solid tumor response to therapy,[66] and it mainly incorporates the size of the tumor and pathologic lymph nodes into its assessment.[67] Unfortunately, RECIST does not always accurately assess the tumor cellular response for STS.[4,66,68,69] This is likely due to the fact that, following radiation, there may be a considerable degree of tumor necrosis without a significant change in size. Alternative guidelines for assessing

Table 1
Imaging modalities and their utility in soft tissue sarcomas

Imaging Modality	Benefits	Limitations	Utility
Plain radiograph	• Identify patterns of calcification and ossification • Low cost	• Inadequate for anatomic surgical planning	• Initial workup
Ultrasound	• No radiation exposure • Can identify vascularity	• Operator dependent • Less useful for deep tumors due to limited tissue penetration	• Initial workup • Image-guided biopsy • Postoperative surveillance
Computed tomography	• Can identify vascular involvement • Distinguishes between cystic and solid tumors	• High radiation exposure • Low contrast resolution	• Initial workup if MRI contra-indicated • Image-guided biopsy • Postoperative surveillance
Magnetic resonance Imaging	• Low radiation exposure • Demonstrates tumor relationship to vasculature, nerves, and bones • T1, T2, and DWI characteristics can point to specific pathologic diagnoses	• Can be contraindicated based on patient factors (ie, metal implants, pacemakers)	• Initial workup: imaging modality of choice
18FDG-PET-CT	• Can identify increased metabolic activity in lymph nodes	• High radiation exposure • Unable to distinguish the residual disease from expected postsurgical changes	• Monitoring response to treatment

tumor response to treatment have emerged; most notably the Choi criteria, which assess both change in tumor size and contrast enhancement on CT and MRI.[70] Additionally, a study by Evilevitch and colleagues[66] in 2008 found that measuring changes in tumor FDG uptake on [18]FDG-PET-CT was significantly more accurate than the RECIST criteria in determining tumor response to therapy, likely reflecting the fact that responses at a cellular level may occur earlier than any observed decrease in size.[4]

SUMMARY

STSs are rare and heterogeneous malignancies. Various imaging modalities can be used in the diagnosis, evaluation, and surveillance of STS. **Table 1** summarizes the benefits, limitations, and utility of each imaging study. The choice of workup and evaluation imaging modality is ultimately dependent on patient and tumor factors and typically requires a multidisciplinary team for proper treatment and surgical planning.

CLINICS CARE POINTS

- Ultrasound findings of a soft tissue mass including increased vascularity, heterogeneity, and size >3cm can be worrisome for sarcoma and should prompt further evaluation with magnetic resonance imaging (MRI).
- MRI should be routinely performed on soft tissue masses prior to resection, unless ultrasound findings clearly identify the mass as a benign lipoma or peripheral nerve sheath tumor.-Staging of a sarcoma should include Computed Tomography (CT) of the chest due to the propensity for pulmonary metastases.
- The role of Positron Emission Tomography CT (PET-CT) in soft tissue sarcoma is generally limited, and its use is primarily in determining response to therapy.

REFERENCES

1. Simon MA, Finn HA. Diagnostic strategy for bone and soft-tissue tumors. J Bone Joint Surg Am 1993;75(4):622–31.
2. Aga P, Singh R, Parihar A, et al. Imaging spectrum in soft tissue sarcomas. Indian J Surg Oncol 2011;2(4):271–9.
3. Wu JS, Hochman MG. Soft-tissue tumors and tumorlike lesions: a systematic imaging approach. Radiology 2009;253(2):297–316.
4. Patel DB, Matcuk GR. Imaging of soft tissue sarcomas. Chin Clin Oncol 2018; 7(4):35.
5. Murray JA. Synovial sarcoma. Orthop Clin North Am 1977;8(4):963–72.
6. Wilkerson BW, Crim JR, Hung M, et al. Characterization of synovial sarcoma calcification. AJR Am J Roentgenol 2012;199(6):W730–4.
7. Banks KP, Bui-Mansfield LT, Chew FS, et al. A compartmental approach to the radiographic evaluation of soft-tissue calcifications. Semin Roentgenol 2005; 40(4):391–407.
8. Amini B, Jessop AC, Ganeshan DM, et al. Contemporary imaging of soft tissue sarcomas. J Surg Oncol 2015;111(5):496–503.
9. Belli P, Costantini M, Mirk P, et al. Role of color Doppler sonography in the assessment of musculoskeletal soft tissue masses. J Ultrasound Med 2000;19(12): 823–30.

10. Carra BJ, Bui-Mansfield LT, O'Brien SD, et al. Sonography of musculoskeletal soft-tissue masses: techniques, pearls, and pitfalls. AJR Am J Roentgenol 2014;202(6):1281–90.
11. Niimi R, Matsumine A, Kusuzaki K, et al. Soft-tissue sarcoma mimicking large haematoma: a report of two cases and review of the literature. J Orthop Surg (Hong Kong) 2006;14(1):90–5.
12. Rougraff BT, Aboulafia A, Biermann JS, et al. Biopsy of soft tissue masses: evidence-based medicine for the musculoskeletal tumor society. Clin Orthop Relat Res 2009;467(11):2783–91.
13. Sundaram M, McGuire MH, Herbold DR. Magnetic resonance imaging of soft tissue masses: an evaluation of fifty-three histologically proven tumors. Magn Reson Imaging 1988;6(3):237–48.
14. Roberts CC, Kransdorf MJ, Beaman FD, et al. ACR appropriateness criteria follow-up of malignant or aggressive musculoskeletal tumors. J Am Coll Radiol 2016;13(4):389–400.
15. Hogeboom WR, Hoekstra HJ, Mooyaart EL, et al. MRI and CT in the preoperative evaluation of soft-tissue tumors. Arch Orthop Trauma Surg 1991;110(3):162–4.
16. Aisen AM, Martel W, Braunstein EM, et al. MRI and CT evaluation of primary bone and soft-tissue tumors. AJR Am J Roentgenol 1986;146(4):749–56.
17. Demas BE, Heelan RT, Lane J, et al. Soft-tissue sarcomas of the extremities: comparison of MR and CT in determining the extent of disease. AJR Am J Roentgenol 1988;150(3):615–20.
18. Hanna SL, Fletcher BD. MR imaging of malignant soft-tissue tumors. Magn Reson Imaging Clin N Am 1995;3(4):629–50.
19. Messiou C, Moskovic E, Vanel D, et al. Primary retroperitoneal soft tissue sarcoma: Imaging appearances, pitfalls and diagnostic algorithm. Eur J Surg Oncol 2017;43(7):1191–8.
20. Lee SY, Jee WH, Jung JY, et al. Differentiation of malignant from benign soft tissue tumours: use of additive qualitative and quantitative diffusion-weighted MR imaging to standard MR imaging at 3.0 T. Eur Radiol 2016;26(3):743–54.
21. Nagata S, Nishimura H, Uchida M, et al. Diffusion-weighted imaging of soft tissue tumors: usefulness of the apparent diffusion coefficient for differential diagnosis. Radiat Med 2008;26(5):287–95.
22. Miwa S, Otsuka T. Practical use of imaging technique for management of bone and soft tissue tumors. J Orthop Sci 2017;22(3):391–400.
23. Verstraete KL, Lang P. Bone and soft tissue tumors: the role of contrast agents for MR imaging. Eur J Radiol 2000;34(3):229–46.
24. De Schepper AM, Ramon FA, Degryse HR. Statistical analysis of MRI parameters predicting malignancy in 141 soft tissue masses. Rofo 1992;156(6):587–91.
25. Gaskin CM, Helms CA. Lipomas, lipoma variants, and well-differentiated liposarcomas (atypical lipomas): results of MRI evaluations of 126 consecutive fatty masses. AJR Am J Roentgenol 2004;182(3):733–9.
26. De La Hoz Polo M, Dick E, Bhumbra R, et al. Surgical considerations when reporting MRI studies of soft tissue sarcoma of the limbs. Skeletal Radiol 2017;46(12):1667–78.
27. Kransdorf MJ, Murphey MD, Wessell DE, et al. ACR Appropriateness Criteria. J Am Coll Radiol 2018;15(5S):S189–97.
28. Panicek DM, Gatsonis C, Rosenthal DI, et al. CT and MR imaging in the local staging of primary malignant musculoskeletal neoplasms: Report of the Radiology Diagnostic Oncology Group. Radiology 1997;202(1):237–46.

29. Subhawong TK, Fishman EK, Swart JE, et al. Soft-tissue masses and masslike conditions: what does CT add to diagnosis and management? AJR Am J Roentgenol 2010;194(6):1559–67.

30. Li Y, Zheng Y, Lin J, et al. Evaluation of the relationship between extremity soft tissue sarcomas and adjacent major vessels using contrast-enhanced multidetector CT and three-dimensional volume-rendered CT angiography: a preliminary study. Acta Radiol 2013;54(8):966–72.

31. Ioannidis JP, Lau J. 18F-FDG PET for the diagnosis and grading of soft-tissue sarcoma: a meta-analysis. J Nucl Med 2003;44(5):717–24.

32. Folpe AL, Lyles RH, Sprouse JT, et al. (F-18) fluorodeoxyglucose positron emission tomography as a predictor of pathologic grade and other prognostic variables in bone and soft tissue sarcoma. Clin Cancer Res 2000;6(4):1279–87.

33. Eary JF, O'Sullivan F, O'Sullivan J, et al. Spatial heterogeneity in sarcoma 18F-FDG uptake as a predictor of patient outcome. J Nucl Med 2008;49(12):1973–9.

34. Eary JF, O'Sullivan F, Powitan Y, et al. Sarcoma tumor FDG uptake measured by PET and patient outcome: a retrospective analysis. Eur J Nucl Med Mol Imaging 2002;29(9):1149–54.

35. Heslin MJ, Lewis JJ, Woodruff JM, et al. Core needle biopsy for diagnosis of extremity soft tissue sarcoma. Ann Surg Oncol 1997;4(5):425–31.

36. Strauss DC, Qureshi YA, Hayes AJ, et al. The role of core needle biopsy in the diagnosis of suspected soft tissue tumours. J Surg Oncol 2010;102(5):523–9.

37. Manaster BJ. Soft-tissue masses: optimal imaging protocol and reporting. AJR Am J Roentgenol 2013;201(3):505–14.

38. Pollock R, Maki R. Introduction to soft tissue sarcoma. In: Amin MB, editor. AJCC cancer staging manual. 8th ed. Chicago: AJCC; 2017. p. 489.

39. Group EESNW. Soft tissue and visceral sarcomas: ESMO Clinical Practice Guidelines for diagnosis, treatment and follow-up. Ann Oncol 2014;25(Suppl 3): iii102–12.

40. Mohammed TL, Chowdhry A, Reddy GP, et al. ACR Appropriateness Criteria® screening for pulmonary metastases. J Thorac Imaging 2011;26(1):W1–3.

41. National Comprehensive Cancer Network (NCCN). NCCN clinical practice guidelines in oncology. Available at;. https://www.nccn.org/professionals/physician_gls. Accessed November 09.

42. Gaballah AH, Jensen CT, Palmquist S, et al. Angiosarcoma: clinical and imaging features from head to toe. Br J Radiol 2017;90(1075):20170039.

43. Thway K, Jones RL, Noujaim J, et al. Epithelioid sarcoma: diagnostic features and genetics. Adv Anat Pathol 2016;23(1):41–9.

44. Ibrahim RM, Steenstrup Jensen S, Juel J. Clear cell sarcoma-A review. J Orthop 2018;15(4):963–6.

45. Ecker BL, Peters MG, McMillan MT, et al. Implications of Lymph Node Evaluation in the Management of Resectable Soft Tissue Sarcoma. Ann Surg Oncol 2017; 24(2):425–33.

46. Asano N, Susa M, Hosaka S, et al. Metastatic patterns of myxoid/round cell liposarcoma: a review of a 25-year experience. Sarcoma 2012;2012:345161.

47. Smolle MA, Leithner A, Bernhardt GA. Abdominal metastases of primary extremity soft tissue sarcoma: A systematic review. World J Clin Oncol 2020;11(2): 74–82.

48. von Mehren M, Kane JM, Bui MM, et al. NCCN guidelines insights: soft tissue sarcoma, version 1.2021. J Natl Compr Canc Netw 2020;18(12):1604–12.

49. Wagner LM, Kremer N, Gelfand MJ, et al. Detection of lymph node metastases in pediatric and adolescent/young adult sarcoma: Sentinel lymph node biopsy

versus fludeoxyglucose positron emission tomography imaging-A prospective trial. Cancer 2017;123(1):155–60.

50. Lucas JD, O'Doherty MJ, Wong JC, et al. Evaluation of fluorodeoxyglucose positron emission tomography in the management of soft-tissue sarcomas. J Bone Joint Surg Br 1998;80(3):441–7.

51. Iagaru A, Chawla S, Menendez L, et al. 18F-FDG PET and PET/CT for detection of pulmonary metastases from musculoskeletal sarcomas. Nucl Med Commun 2006;27(10):795–802.

52. Roberge D, Hickeson M, Charest M, et al. Initial McGill experience with fluorodeoxyglucose pet/ct staging of soft-tissue sarcoma. Curr Oncol 2010;17(6): 18–22.

53. Sood S, Baheti AD, Shinagare AB, et al. Imaging features of primary and metastatic alveolar soft part sarcoma: single institute experience in 25 patients. Br J Radiol 2014;87(1036):20130719.

54. Dim DC, Cooley LD, Miranda RN. Clear cell sarcoma of tendons and aponeuroses: a review. Arch Pathol Lab Med 2007;131(1):152–6.

55. Shweikeh F, Bukavina L, Saeed K, et al. Brain metastasis in bone and soft tissue cancers: a review of incidence, interventions, and outcomes. Sarcoma 2014; 2014:475175.

56. von Mehren M, Lor Randall R, DeLaney T, et al. NCCN Clinical practice Guidelines in Oncology (NCCN Guidelines) Soft Tissue Sarcoma. 2014. p. 126.

57. Schwab JH, Boland PJ, Antonescu C, et al. Spinal metastases from myxoid liposarcoma warrant screening with magnetic resonance imaging. Cancer 2007; 110(8):1815–22.

58. Schwab JH, Boland P, Guo T, et al. Skeletal metastases in myxoid liposarcoma: an unusual pattern of distant spread. Ann Surg Oncol 2007;14(4):1507–14.

59. Tateishi U, Hasegawa T, Beppu Y, et al. Prognostic significance of MRI findings in patients with myxoid-round cell liposarcoma. AJR Am J Roentgenol 2004;182(3): 725–31.

60. Whooley BP, Mooney MM, Gibbs JF, et al. Effective follow-up strategies in soft tissue sarcoma. Semin Surg Oncol 1999;17(1):83–7.

61. Whooley BP, Gibbs JF, Mooney MM, et al. Primary extremity sarcoma: what is the appropriate follow-up? Ann Surg Oncol 2000;7(1):9–14.

62. Kane JM. Surveillance strategies for patients following surgical resection of soft tissue sarcomas. Curr Opin Oncol 2004;16(4):328–32.

63. Choi H, Varma DG, Fornage BD, et al. Soft-tissue sarcoma: MR imaging vs sonography for detection of local recurrence after surgery. AJR Am J Roentgenol 1991;157(2):353–8.

64. Arya S, Nagarkatti DG, Dudhat SB, et al. Soft tissue sarcomas: ultrasonographic evaluation of local recurrences. Clin Radiol 2000;55(3):193–7.

65. Park SY, Chung HW, Chae SY, et al. Comparison of MRI and PET-CT in detecting the loco-regional recurrence of soft tissue sarcomas during surveillance. Skeletal Radiol 2016;45(10):1375–84.

66. Evilevitch V, Weber WA, Tap WD, et al. Reduction of glucose metabolic activity is more accurate than change in size at predicting histopathologic response to neoadjuvant therapy in high-grade soft-tissue sarcomas. Clin Cancer Res 2008; 14(3):715–20.

67. Eisenhauer EA, Therasse P, Bogaerts J, et al. New response evaluation criteria in solid tumours: revised RECIST guideline (version 1.1). Eur J Cancer 2009;45(2): 228–47.

68. Tuma RS. Sometimes size doesn't matter: reevaluating RECIST and tumor response rate endpoints. J Natl Cancer Inst 2006;98(18):1272–4.
69. Gehan EA, Tefft MC. Will there be resistance to the RECIST (Response Evaluation Criteria in Solid Tumors)? J Natl Cancer Inst 2000;92(3):179–81.
70. Stacchiotti S, Verderio P, Messina A, et al. Tumor response assessment by modified Choi criteria in localized high-risk soft tissue sarcoma treated with chemotherapy. Cancer 2012;118(23):5857–66.

Wide Resection of Extremity/Truncal Soft Tissue Sarcomas

Ankit Patel, MD, John M. Kane III, MD*

KEYWORDS

• Sarcoma • Wide resection • Margins • Local recurrence • Amputation

KEY POINTS

• The potentially curative treatment of a primary soft tissue sarcoma is negative margin wide resection.
• The planned surgical resection should include the clinical tumor (defined by physical examination and staging imaging) as well as an en bloc margin of at least 1 to 2 cm of grossly uninvolved tissues but can be less for oncologically equivalent barrier structures (fascia, periosteum, and so forth) or to preserve an adjacent critical structure.
• The role of radiation and/or chemotherapy as part of multimodality treatment should be discussed in a multidisciplinary setting before proceeding with surgery, as there can be potential benefits to a neoadjuvant (preoperative) approach.
• An isolated local recurrence is still potentially curable and should be addressed in a manner similar to a primary sarcoma, including the possibility of radiation/reirradiation and/or chemotherapy.
• Amputation for an extremity sarcoma is rarely necessary and should only be performed after other limb salvage treatment options have been considered.

INTRODUCTION

In the absence of distant metastatic disease, the potentially curative treatment of a primary soft tissue sarcoma is surgical wide resection. The principal goal of wide resection is to obtain long-term local control. A soft tissue sarcoma often has a "pseudocapsule" with extension of microscopic tumor cells outside of the clinically visible portions of the primary tumor. Surgical wide resection needs to fully encompass cells outside of the pseudocapsule by including surrounding normal tissues. In the ideal situation, wide resection should result in pathologically negative surgical margins. When wide resection will not include microscopic tumor cells, adjacent critical

Department of Surgical Oncology, Roswell Park Comprehensive Cancer Center, Elm and Carlton Streets, Buffalo, NY 14263, USA
* Corresponding author.
E-mail address: john.kane@roswellpark.org

Surg Clin N Am 102 (2022) 551–565
https://doi.org/10.1016/j.suc.2022.05.002   surgical.theclinics.com
0039-6109/22/© 2022 Elsevier Inc. All rights reserved.

structures (major blood vessels, nerves, bony structures) or obtaining negative margins would result in significant morbidity such as amputation, consideration should be given to the addition of radiation therapy to improve local control.

Another important surgical consideration for the treatment of soft tissue sarcomas is the high implantation potential. Similar to a carcinoma, disseminated microscopic sarcoma cells have the ability to remain viable within the prior surgical field (biopsy sites, the wide resection scar, and so forth). Therefore, every effort should be made to avoid violating the gross tumor at the time of surgical resection. Similarly, thoughtful planning of the original preoperative diagnostic biopsy is helpful to ideally allow for en bloc excision of the prior biopsy site as part of the formal wide resection. In general, incisional biopsies have been associated with an increased risk for both biopsy tract contamination and local recurrence.[1] In the era of multimodality therapy, especially with the utilization of radiation, excision of a prior core needle biopsy tract en bloc with the wide resection specimen likely has less of an impact on local recurrence.[2] Core needle biopsy site excision should still be considered if technically possible with minimal morbidity.

Before the 1980s, extremity soft tissue sarcomas were treated with amputation. Although one might assume that this was due to the limitations of radiation therapy at that time, the primary reason was actually a lack of precise 3-dimensional imaging techniques. Without an ability to preoperatively define whether an extremity sarcoma simply abutted or encased critical structures, amputation was the only surgical approach that would likely result in negative surgical margins. A seminal study at the National Cancer Institute published in 1982 showed that, although local recurrences were higher for limb-sparing surgery versus amputation (15% vs 0%, respectively, $P = 0.06$), there was no difference in 5-year overall survival (83% vs 88%, respectively, $P = 0.99$).[3] These results ushered in the era of multimodality limb salvage surgery for extremity sarcomas.

PREOPERATIVE CONSIDERATIONS
Staging Imaging for Wide Resection Planning

The purpose of preoperative imaging is to allow for precise surgical planning by defining the relationship of the sarcoma to adjacent anatomic structures: skin, muscle, blood vessels, major nerves, and bone. Soft tissue sarcomas that abut a critical structure can still undergo wide resection with anticipated close or microscopically positive margins, but surgery may need to be combined with radiation. Alternatively, sarcomas that encase a critical structure will require either resection/potential reconstruction of the involved structure or consideration for amputation if it is an extremity soft tissue sarcoma.

Although some soft tissue sarcomas have a rim of surrounding edema on imaging, there are limited data supporting that the edema consistently contains microscopic tumor cells and should be included as part of the "tumor target" for wide resection.[4,5] However, myxofibrosarcoma and undifferentiated pleomorphic sarcoma (UPS) frequently have an infiltrative growth pattern. On MRI, this can appear as surrounding edema that actually contains extensive tumor extension, known as a "tail sign."[6] This finding is illustrated in **Fig. 1**. Consequently, adequate staging imaging is critical to the surgical planning of the oncologically appropriate wide resection. In general, ultrasound will not provide adequate information for wide resection planning except for very small, superficial sarcomas. Contrast-enhanced CT scan will frequently provide appropriate imaging of the primary sarcoma, including the relationship to surrounding anatomic structures. For certain histologies that have either an infiltrative or a myxoid component (myxoid liposarcoma, myxofibrosarcoma, fibromyxoid sarcoma, UPS),

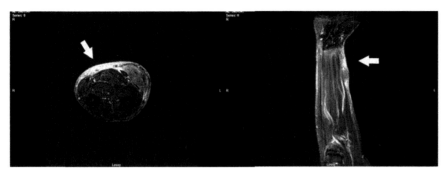

Fig. 1. MRI showing the "edema" surrounding a forearm myxofibrosarcoma that actually represents infiltrative tumor extension, known as the "tail sign" (*arrows*).

MRI can better define the extent of the local tumor. Imaging of soft tissue sarcomas is discussed extensively in the corresponding article on this subject.

Sequencing of Multimodality Therapy with Wide Resection

Radiation
Factors associated with an increased risk for local recurrence following sarcoma wide resection include tumor size, higher grade, and certain histologies.[7] In addition, a very powerful predictor for local recurrence is inadequate resection margins.[7,8] If pathologically negative margins are not technically possible with wide resection, consideration should be given to the addition of radiation therapy to surgery. This topic is discussed in great detail in the article on radiation. Preoperative anticipation of the likelihood of obtaining negative margins with the proposed surgery also helps to determine the sequencing of any radiation therapy. A potential role for radiation is not simply based on the risk of local recurrence. The potential morbidity of a future local recurrence should also factor into the decision-making process. A negative margin wide resection may likely be technically possible for a large, high-grade sarcoma of the superficial buttock. Furthermore, any future local recurrence would be associated with low morbidity if additional resection was necessary. In this situation, the sequencing of treatment would likely be wide resection alone, reserving possible adjuvant radiation therapy only for an unanticipated microscopically positive surgical margin. Alternatively, a large, high-grade sarcoma of the posterior compartment of the thigh abutting the femur and sciatic nerve will not be amenable to a negative margin wide resection short of amputation. In addition, a local recurrence could be very morbid, potentially requiring amputation. In this situation, the plan would be to pursue preoperative radiation therapy followed by surgical wide resection.

In general, if there is a strong clinical indication for radiation, preoperative radiation is favored unless the negative impact on postoperative wound healing would be significant. When preoperative radiation is used, there is a well-defined tumor target for treatment planning, a smaller treatment field, and a lower radiation dose can be administered owing to the well-oxygenated tumor. For extremity sarcomas, a randomized, prospective study noted that the lower radiation dose and smaller field size associated with preoperative radiation correlate with improved long-term functionality of the extremity (fibrosis, joint stiffness, edema, range of motion).[9] The downside of preoperative radiation is the adverse impact on wound healing. The National Cancer Institute of Canada randomized, prospective trial of preoperative versus postoperative radiation for extremity sarcomas showed that preoperative radiation essentially doubled the rate of postoperative wound healing complications (35%) as compared with surgery alone (17%).[10] This negative effect was most pronounced for the lower extremity. Therefore, if preoperative radiation is going to be considered, preoperative planning of the anticipated approach to wound closure of the surgical defect is critical, including involvement of plastic surgery for the potential use of vascularized, unirradiated tissue. This topic is covered nicely in the article on reconstruction. Finally, if it is unclear if radiation will be necessary as part of the multimodality treatment of the sarcoma, then the decision regarding potential radiation should be deferred to the postoperative setting, based on the margin status on the final pathology. The pros and cons of preoperative versus postoperative radiation are reviewed in the radiation article.

Chemotherapy

Many soft tissue sarcomas, especially high-grade tumors and certain histologies, will have a high risk for distant metastases. Given the rarity of sarcomas combined with the fact that there are probably 100 different histologic subtypes (each with slightly different biologic behaviors), it has been very difficult to perform large, prospective, randomized studies of chemotherapy. Consequently, the overall benefit of chemotherapy as part of the multimodality treatment of soft tissue sarcomas is not as well defined as for other malignancies (colorectal cancer, breast cancer). In general, chemotherapy is considered for otherwise healthy patients at "high risk" for developing hematogenous metastatic disease.

Early adjuvant chemotherapy data suggested an improvement in both local control and overall survival.[11] The original as well as an updated meta-analysis of the available adjuvant chemotherapy literature noted an absolute benefit of 3% to 6% for local recurrence and 4% to 11% for overall survival.[12,13] Unfortunately, some modern adjuvant chemotherapy trials have failed to show a durable, statistically significant survival benefit.[14,15] Traditionally, patients with high-risk sarcomas received 4 to 6 cycles of adjuvant chemotherapy. Although there might be some variation based on specific histologies, the most common chemotherapy regimens used for sarcomas are anthracycline-based (doxorubicin or epirubicin), typically with the addition of ifosfamide.

Other sarcoma clinical trials have focused on more limited cycles of neoadjuvant chemotherapy approach (ie, before surgery). The potential benefits of neoadjuvant chemotherapy are treating subclinical micrometastatic disease as early as possible and using the primary tumor as an "in vivo" marker of treatment response. A complete pathologic response to sarcoma neoadjuvant therapy has correlated with improved overall survival.[16] Downstaging of a large sarcoma following neoadjuvant chemotherapy could facilitate the subsequent wide resection. More importantly, a response to neoadjuvant therapy by the primary tumor would justify ongoing treatment with that regimen (including the associated morbidity). Alternatively, if the primary tumor does not respond after 2 to 3 cycles of neoadjuvant chemotherapy, then additional treatment with an ineffective regimen can be avoided. Finally, the development of clinical distant metastatic disease during neoadjuvant chemotherapy (essentially synchronous metastases) spares the patient from the morbidity of what would have been a noncurative surgery.

More recent sarcoma studies have shown that overall survival with 3 cycles of neoadjuvant chemotherapy is noninferior to 3 cycles of neoadjuvant with an additional 2 cycles of postoperative chemotherapy and that standard anthracycline/ifosfamide neoadjuvant chemotherapy is equivalent to specific histology-tailored chemotherapy regimens.[17,18] Similar to adjuvant chemotherapy, a randomized neoadjuvant chemotherapy trial did not show a statistically significant improvement in overall survival.[19]

When trying to assess for any potential survival benefit from either adjuvant or neoadjuvant chemotherapy, one issue is that "high risk" in many clinical trials was not precisely defined (often only size, grade, and depth criteria), representing a fairly broad range of true metastatic risk. The Sarculator is a nomogram for both primary and recurrent sarcomas that incorporates both age and tumor size (as continuous variables) as well as grade and specific histology to predict distant metastases and overall survival.[20] This nomogram has been validated across fairly large, diverse sarcoma patient populations.[21,22] Although a previous European Organisation for Research and Treatment of Cancer randomized trial of surgery alone versus the addition of 5 cycles of adjuvant doxorubicin/ifosfamide chemotherapy failed to show a survival benefit for chemotherapy, the results were reanalyzed using the Sarculator to more precisely categorize the participants' predicted overall survival.[23] For lower-risk patients with a greater than 60% predicted overall survival, there was no observed benefit to adjuvant chemotherapy. In contrast, for patients defined as high risk (Sarculator predicted overall survival <60%), adjuvant chemotherapy significantly reduced the risk of dying (hazard ratio = 0.50; 95% confidence interval, 0.30–0.90). A separate analysis of the previously mentioned study of neoadjuvant anthracycline/ifosfamide chemotherapy versus histology-specific chemotherapy noted similar findings; the observed overall survival of patients who received neoadjuvant anthracycline/ifosfamide chemotherapy was significantly better than the Sarculator-predicted survival if they were defined as high risk (a predicted overall survival of <60%).[24] This perceived chemotherapy benefit was not seen for a Sarculator predicted overall survival of greater than 60%. In conclusion, when considering the role of chemotherapy, "high risk" should probably be defined as at least a 40% chance for developing metastatic disease.

OPERATIVE TECHNIQUE
Margin Planning

The goal of surgical wide resection is to obtain microscopically negative margins (R0), if technically possible without excessive morbidity, while avoiding tumor spillage into the surgical field. If the intent is to have a planned microscopically positive margin (R1) on a critical structure (major nerve, blood vessel, bone) for limb preservation or to reduce surgical morbidity, wide resection should still strive to resect all gross tumor. One study has shown that the risk for local recurrence following a planned microscopically positive margin on a critical structure is much lower than for an unplanned positive margin (3.6% vs 37.5%, respectively).[25] Therefore, a planned microscopically positive margin at a specific critical location does not mean that the status of the remainder of the margins does not matter.

When planning the extent of the wide resection in terms of margin distance, the tumor target is defined by physical examination as well as correlating the preoperative staging imaging with anatomic landmarks. Different tissue types are variably penetrated by the microscopic tumor cells outside of the sarcoma pseudocapsule. Skin, fat, and muscle are more readily invaded by tumor extension. In contrast, fascia and periosteum are excellent "oncologic" barrier structures. Therefore, although the general dogma is to obtain at least 1 cm (ideally, 2 cm) of uninvolved normal tissues around the clinical sarcoma at the time of surgery, only a few millimeters of a barrier structure (such as fascia) are adequate for an oncologically appropriate resection.

Additional Technical Considerations

- Soft tissue sarcomas have high implantation potential. If technically possible, the previous biopsy site (especially an incisional biopsy) should be incorporated into the wide resection specimen.

- Given that fascia is an excellent oncologic barrier to tumor penetration, for sarcomas located within a defined anatomic compartment, an attempt should be made to not violate uninvolved adjacent compartments at the time of wide resection. An exception would be if the intercompartmental fascia needs to be resected en bloc as one of the oncologic margins.
- Unless directly invaded or encased, critical structures (such as major nerves, blood vessels, and bone) can typically be preserved. Dissection just inside the epineurium can often preserve the nerve. Excision of small portions of adventitia may allow for vascular preservation. For sarcomas directly adjacent to bone, resection of a portion of en bloc periosteum is an appropriate oncologic margin.
- Resection of clinically significant arteries and veins is oncologically appropriate in the setting of function preservation. Major peripheral veins are usually not reconstructed owing to very low patency rates. A decision regarding prosthetic versus biologic arterial reconstruction should be based on additional factors, such as radiation, infection risk, and the available defect reconstruction options.
- Especially in the setting of preoperative radiation, biologic material reconstruction of abdominal wall wide resection defects is favored over prosthetic mesh. For biologic material reconstruction, it is critical to cover the material with well-vascularized tissue to allow for incorporation.
- The orientation of the specimen should be precisely marked for pathology in at least 2 perpendicular planes. The anticipated closest clinical margin should also be identified for focused pathologic assessment. Ideally, the specimen should be hand carried to the pathology gross room so that the surgeon can directly convey the anatomic location and the exact orientation of the specimen.
- As many of the resected tissues significantly retract when divided, especially muscle, the intraoperative clinical margins (1–2 cm of grossly normal tissue) do not always precisely correlate with the margin distances on the final pathology. There is also specimen shrinkage in formalin. In essence, the final pathology margins are often closer to the tumor than what was observed clinically at the time of surgery.
- The periphery of the wide resection field should be marked with metallic clips to act as fiducials for any postoperative radiation treatment planning as well as to define the surgical bed on future surveillance imaging studies.
- Surgical drains should be placed within any anticipated soft tissue defect in the wide resection field. The exit site for a drain should be very close to the wide resection incision so that it is included within any postoperative radiation field or can easily be excised if there is a future local recurrence.
- Postoperative seromas or hematomas can negatively impact wound healing, and their ongoing evolution over time can complicate postoperative radiation treatment planning. Therefore, drains should remain in place until the associated soft tissue defect is completely obliterated. In the setting of preoperative radiation, this could often be several weeks.

SPECIFIC SITUATIONS
Accidental Intraoperative Tumor Spillage

Because of the high implantation potential of soft tissue sarcomas, intraoperative tumor spillage will theoretically contaminate the entire surgical field with microscopic tumor cells. If technically possible, the first salvage approach would be to completely close the original incision, reprepare the surgical field, and approach the sarcoma wide resection via a new separate incision that would also encompass the original incision/surgical field as part of the specimen. If a new second incision approach is not technically possible, then an attempt should be made to close the defect in the tumor capsule, resect an additional margin of normal tissue adjacent to the area of violation, and copiously irrigate the surgical field (consider sterile water) once the specimen is removed. Intraoperative tumor spillage could also contribute to a potential decision to pursue adjuvant radiation.

Superficial Sarcomas

Except for the head and neck location, wide resection of a superficial sarcoma can be fairly straightforward from a technical standpoint. If the sarcoma is several centimeters away from the skin surface, then a wide resection can be approached via a more traditional surgical incision with skin flaps. However, if the sarcoma is close to the skin (<2 cm), then an appropriate portion of overlying skin should be resected en bloc with the specimen. Radial margins would include 2 cm of normal-appearing subcutaneous fat around the sarcoma. Similar to the skin, if a superficial sarcoma is several centimeters from the underlying fascia, then the deep margin can be an appropriate amount of subcutaneous fat. Conversely, if the sarcoma is close to the fascia, then the fascia should be resected as the en bloc deep margin (**Fig. 2**)

Although there can be a tendency to consider complex reconstructions for a superficial sarcoma wide resection defect, in most situations, simple is better. This is to minimize potential contamination of the reconstruction donor site with microscopic tumor cells. If there are exposed underlying critical structures or postoperative radiation is likely, then consideration can be given to rotation flaps or other reconstruction approaches. Otherwise, if the wide resection bed is muscle, a split-thickness skin graft or healing by secondary intention is an appropriate option. Unique situations, such as coverage of exposed tendon or devascularized bone, are discussed in the plastic surgery reconstruction article.

As previously noted, myxofibrosarcoma is a histology with a propensity for extensive subcutaneous extension along fascial planes for significant distances. If this unique growth pattern is not appreciated, standard sarcoma wide resection margins will almost certainly result in positive margins on the final pathology with a very high risk for subsequent local recurrence. For myxofibrosarcoma, the wide resection margins should be measured out from the radiographic extent of the tumor, correlated with anatomic landmarks. Consideration should also be given to delayed reconstruction, leaving the wide resection defect open pending confirmation of negative margins on the final pathology. This approach, incorporating temporizing negative pressure therapy (wound vacuum-assisted closure), has been associated with a significantly lower risk for subsequent local recurrence.[26]

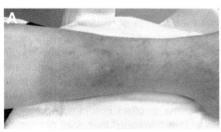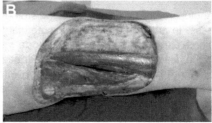

Fig. 2. Wide resection of a lower leg superficial sarcoma requiring excision of the fascia as the en bloc deep margin. (*A*) Before resection (following preoperative radiation). (*B*) The wide resection surgical defect.

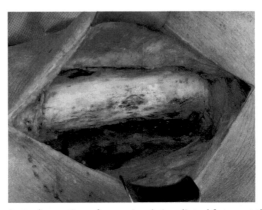

Fig. 3. Extensive periosteal resection of a previously irradiated femur at the time of sarcoma wide resection.

Periosteal Resection

Periosteum is an excellent oncologic barrier to sarcoma penetration. For a sarcoma directly abutting or adherent to an adjacent bone, the periosteum in that area should be resected as the en bloc margin. Small periosteal defects that will be covered with well-vascularized tissue are unlikely to compromise the integrity of the bone. Alternatively, a large area of periosteal stripping of a weight-bearing bone (such as the femur) is associated with a risk for fracture (**Fig. 3**). Fracture risk is further increased with the use of radiation therapy. The rate of nonunion and other negative issues with healing is fairly high in this situation. The reported risk for radiation-associated femur fracture is approximately 1% to 9% with an increased odds ratio of 3.5 to 22.7 for periosteal stripping greater than 10 to 20 cm.[27,28] Intensity-modulated radiation therapy has been associated with a lower risk for fracture, likely because of the decreased circumferential radiation dose to the femur.[29] For extensive periosteal stripping (especially with radiation), prophylactic intramedullary nailing to reduce the risk for fracture should be considered, often at a separate surgical setting. For sarcomas of the scalp, resection of the adjacent skull periosteum will preclude direct split-thickness skin graft coverage. An alternative option to complex flap reconstruction would be placement of Integra bilayer dermal template (sometimes requiring burring of the skull outer table to provide access to the vascularized diploic space) followed by delayed skin grafting.[30]

Radiation-Associated Angiosarcoma

Angiosarcoma is an aggressive histology with a high rate of distant metastatic disease. In addition, there is the potential for multifocality, discontiguous in-transit lesions, as well as regional lymph node metastases. Angiosarcoma can arise de novo in the head and neck region of older patients or in the setting of chronic lymphedema, but there is also a strong association with prior radiation therapy. In the modern era, the most common scenario is status post prior radiation for the treatment of breast cancer. The clinical presentation of angiosarcoma is often insidious, a yellowish discoloration of the skin, mild edema, or violaceous "bruising" that does not resolve over time (**Fig. 4**). Skin involvement is common, even in the setting of an underlying dominant mass. Consequently, a traditional mastectomy used for breast cancer with preservation of the overlying skin envelope is very unlikely to encompass all of

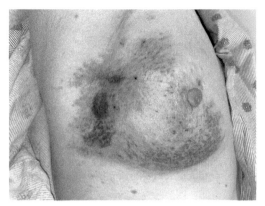

Fig. 4. The classic violaceous "bruising" appearance of a radiation associated angiosarcoma of the breast.

the angiosarcoma. Given the multifocality and potential field defect from the radiation, even a standard wide resection of the clinically apparent tumor with appropriate sarcoma margins is associated with a high risk of local recurrence. Therefore, the recommended approach is a more radical resection: mastectomy plus all previously irradiated skin (**Fig. 5**). In a study by Li and colleagues[31] of 76 women with radiation-associated breast angiosarcoma, both 5-year local recurrence rates and disease-specific survival were significantly better following radical resection as compared with a more conservative wide excision. Secondary to the high risk for developing distant metastases, many patients with radiation-associated breast angiosarcoma will receive neoadjuvant chemotherapy. This can result in a significant, although often transient, clinical response by the visible tumor (**Fig. 6**). However, this clinical "downstaging" does not alter the original planned extent of the radical resection. Therefore, if there is clinical tumor located outside of well-defined anatomic landmarks, adjunct maneuvers to identify these areas at the time of the definitive surgery include pretreatment photographs and India ink tattooing of the periphery of the clinical tumor.

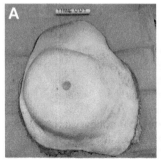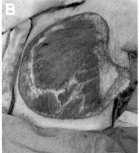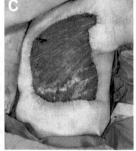

Fig. 5. Radical resection (mastectomy plus all previously irradiated skin) of a radiation associated left breast angiosarcoma. (*A*) Surgical specimen. (*B*) Wide resection defect. (*C*) Surgical defect after skin edge marsupialization but before skin grafting.

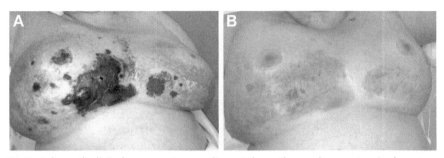

Fig. 6. A dramatic clinical response to neoadjuvant chemotherapy by an extensive breast angiosarcoma. (*A*) Initial presentation. (*B*) Following neoadjuvant chemotherapy.

LOCAL RECURRENCE

Local recurrence rates following multimodality therapy (wide resection and radiation) are expected to be ≤20%, slightly higher in the setting of a planned positive margin for limb salvage.[32] A sarcoma local recurrence is often indicative of a more aggressive tumor biology and is associated with a higher risk for developing distant metastatic disease.[8,33] However, many patients with an isolated local recurrence can still be cured. Consequently, a local recurrence should be addressed in a manner identical to a primary sarcoma. Staging imaging should be performed to assess the extent of the recurrence, any involvement of critical structures, and to rule out metastatic disease. For a very aggressive histologic subtype, especially where "downstaging" would facilitate wide resection, consideration could be given to neoadjuvant chemotherapy. If radiation therapy was not previously administered as part of the treatment of the original sarcoma, local recurrence would be a strong indication for considering radiation. In highly selected cases whereby radiation was previously administered, there can be a role for reirradiation (including proton therapy) with reasonable local control rates.[34,35] However, reirradiation has been associated with increased wound healing complications and morbidity.[34] From a surgical perspective, the proposed wide resection would need to include the local recurrence, ideally with negative margins. For a multifocal local recurrence, the entire prior surgical site may need to be resected (including the surgical scar, drain exit sites, and so forth). Given the complexity of a local recurrence and the potential need for a multimodality therapy approach, these cases should always be discussed in a multidisciplinary setting at a center with expertise in the treatment of sarcomas.

AMPUTATION

Although amputation for extremity soft tissue sarcoma can result in slightly lower local recurrence rates as compared with limb salvage surgery, there is no associated overall survival benefit.[36] In the modern era of multimodality therapy, long-term limb salvage rates, including recurrent tumor, exceed 90%. Consequently, amputation for an extremity sarcoma should be a rare event. Potential indications for amputation include extensive multifocal tumor, invasion/encasement of multiple critical structures (primarily nerves and/or bone), a nonfunctional, severely painful extremity due to advanced local tumor, or multiple patient comorbidities that would preclude a complex wide resection/reconstruction or neoadjuvant chemotherapy for potential downstaging. As noted in the "Operative Technique" section, isolated vascular involvement is not an indication for amputation. Arterial resection/reconstruction should always be

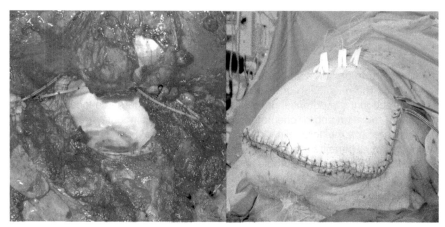

Fig. 7. Placement of perineural infusion catheters for postoperative pain control following a right hip disarticulation.

considered. Although major venous resection can lead to a congested, edematous extremity, it does not typically compromise tissue perfusion. Isolated major nerve involvement can be addressed with nerve grafting techniques or even en bloc nerve resection with either tendon transfer or supportive splints/braces, resulting in a partially functional "bioprosthesis" (such as sciatic nerve resection in the lower extremity). Similar to local recurrence, a patient with an extremity sarcoma potentially facing amputation should be evaluated by a multidisciplinary team at a sarcoma center.

For locally advanced or multifocal sarcomas located distal to the axilla or groin, isolated regional therapy is an additional treatment option for limb preservation. Isolated limb perfusion (ILP) with melphalan and tumor necrosis factor (TNF) has been widely used throughout Europe. Because TNF is not available for clinical use in the United States, the somewhat less invasive isolated limb infusion (ILI) with melphalan and actinomycin D has been the preferred approach. For unresectable extremity sarcomas facing amputation, a meta-analysis of ILP/ILI noted an overall response rate of 73.3%, a complete response rate of 25.8%, and an overall limb salvage rate of 73.8% (median time to local progression 22.1 months).[37]

Historically, amputation for a soft tissue sarcoma was performed at the joint proximal to the tumor. However, given that residual limb length has a direct correlation with functionality, the oncologic principle to obtain negative margins should be applied when determining the appropriate level of amputation. Variations of amputation can also be considered, such an internal hemipelvectomy (with preservation of the extremity) for an iliac fossa sarcoma whereby the iliac vessels and sciatic nerve are not involved. In addition to typical postoperative pain, patients undergoing amputation are at increased risk for phantom sensations and phantom pain. Although the results in the literature are mixed regarding the long-term impact on phantom pain, intraoperative placement of perineural infusion catheters into the amputated nerve stumps can be considered a postoperative pain management adjunct (**Fig. 7**).[38–40]

SUMMARY

The potentially curative treatment of a primary soft tissue sarcoma is negative margin wide resection. The planned surgical resection should include the clinical tumor (defined by physical examination and staging imaging) as well as an en bloc margin of normal surrounding tissue to fully encompass any microscopic tumor outside of the pseudocapsule. Ideal margins are typically at least 1 to 2 cm of grossly uninvolved tissues but can be less for oncologically equivalent barrier structures (fascia, periosteum, and similar) or to preserve an adjacent critical structure. Gross tumor spillage should be avoided. The orientation of the incision and placement of surgical drains should take into account the potential need for future surgery if there is a local recurrence. The role of radiation and/or chemotherapy as part of multimodality treatment should be discussed in a multidisciplinary setting before proceeding with surgery, as there can be potential benefits to a neoadjuvant (preoperative) approach. An isolated local recurrence is still potentially curable and should be addressed in a manner similar to a primary sarcoma, including the possibility of radiation/reirradiation and/or chemotherapy. Amputation for an extremity sarcoma is rarely necessary and should only be performed after other limb salvage treatment options have been considered.

CLINICS CARE POINTS

- The potential roles of radiation and chemotherapy in the multimodality treatment of a soft tissue sarcoma should be discussed before surgery in order to optimize the sequencing of therapies.
- Sarcoma surgical wide resection needs to encompass the clinical tumor as well as an en bloc "oncologically appropriate" margin of surrounding clinically uninvolved tissues.
- Intraoperative tumor spillage should be avoided, as it will contaminate the surgical field with viable sarcoma cells, decreasing the chance for long-term local control.
- Intraoperative maneuvers (such as incision orientation, placement of surgical clips within the periphery of the resection bed, drain exit sites) can positively impact the overall management of a sarcoma.
- Reconstruction options for the anticipated wide resection defect should be determined before surgery. In addition, the oncologically appropriate operation should not be compromised in order to facilitate a less complex reconstruction.
- The management of a sarcoma local recurrence and the potential need for amputation require complex decision making. Those patients are best treated at an institution with multispecialty sarcoma expertise.

DISCLOSURE

None.

REFERENCES

1. Barrientos-Ruiz I, Ortiz-Cruz EJ, Serrano-Montilla J, et al. Are biopsy tracts a concern for seeding and local recurrence in sarcomas? Clin Orthop Relat Res 2017;475(2):511–8.
2. Klein A, Birkenmaier C, Fromm J, et al. Sarcomas of the extremities and the pelvis: comparing local recurrence after incisional and after core-needle biopsy. World J Surg Oncol 2022;20(1):14.
3. Rosenberg SA, Tepper J, Glatstein E, et al. The treatment of soft-tissue sarcomas of the extremities: prospective randomized evaluations of (1) limb-sparing surgery plus radiation therapy compared with amputation and (2) the role of adjuvant chemotherapy. Ann Surg 1982;196(3):305–15.

4. White LM, Wunder JS, Bell RS, et al. Histologic assessment of peritumoral edema in soft tissue sarcoma. Int J Radiat Oncol Biol Phys 2005;61(5):1439–45.

5. Panicek DM, Schwartz LH. Soft tissue edema around musculoskeletal sarcomas at magnetic resonance imaging. Sarcoma 1997;1(3–4):189–91.

6. Yoo HJ, Hong SH, Kang Y, et al. MR imaging of myxofibrosarcoma and undifferentiated sarcoma with emphasis on tail sign; diagnostic and prognostic value. Eur Radiol 2014;24(8):1749–57.

7. Cahlon O, Brennan MF, Jia X, et al. A postoperative nomogram for local recurrence risk in extremity soft tissue sarcomas after limb-sparing surgery without adjuvant radiation. Ann Surg 2012;255(2):343–7.

8. Trovik CS, Bauer HC, Alvegård TA, et al. Surgical margins, local recurrence and metastasis in soft tissue sarcomas: 559 surgically-treated patients from the Scandinavian Sarcoma Group Register. Eur J Cancer 2000;36(6):710–6.

9. Davis AM, O'Sullivan B, Turcotte R, et al. Late radiation morbidity following randomization to preoperative versus postoperative radiotherapy in extremity soft tissue sarcoma. Radiother Oncol 2005;75(1):48–53.

10. O'Sullivan B, Davis AM, Turcotte R, et al. Preoperative versus postoperative radiotherapy in soft-tissue sarcoma of the limbs: a randomised trial. Lancet (London, England) 2002;359(9325):2235–41.

11. Chang AE, Kinsella T, Glatstein E, et al. Adjuvant chemotherapy for patients with high-grade soft-tissue sarcomas of the extremity. J Clin Oncol 1988;6(9): 1491–500.

12. Adjuvant chemotherapy for localised resectable soft-tissue sarcoma of adults: meta-analysis of individual data. Sarcoma Meta-analysis Collaboration. Lancet (London, England) 1997;350(9092):1647–54.

13. Pervaiz N, Colterjohn N, Farrokhyar F, et al. A systematic meta-analysis of randomized controlled trials of adjuvant chemotherapy for localized resectable soft-tissue sarcoma. Cancer 2008;113(3):573–81.

14. Frustaci S, De Paoli A, Bidoli E, et al. Ifosfamide in the adjuvant therapy of soft tissue sarcomas. Oncology 2003;65(Suppl 2):80–4.

15. Woll PJ, Reichardt P, Le Cesne A, et al. Adjuvant chemotherapy with doxorubicin, ifosfamide, and lenograstim for resected soft-tissue sarcoma (EORTC 62931): a multicentre randomised controlled trial. Lancet Oncol 2012;13(10):1045–54.

16. Bonvalot S, Wunder J, Gronchi A, et al. Complete pathological response to neoadjuvant treatment is associated with better survival outcomes in patients with soft tissue sarcoma: Results of a retrospective multicenter study. Eur J Surg Oncol 2021;47(8):2166–72.

17. Gronchi A, Stacchiotti S, Verderio P, et al. Short, full-dose adjuvant chemotherapy (CT) in high-risk adult soft tissue sarcomas (STS): long-term follow-up of a randomized clinical trial from the Italian Sarcoma Group and the Spanish Sarcoma Group. Ann Oncol 2016;27(12):2283–8.

18. Gronchi A, Palmerini E, Quagliuolo V, et al. Neoadjuvant chemotherapy in high-risk soft tissue sarcomas: final results of a randomized trial from Italian (ISG), Spanish (GEIS), French (FSG), and Polish (PSG) Sarcoma groups. J Clin Oncol 2020;38(19):2178–86.

19. Gortzak E, Azzarelli A, Buesa J, et al. A randomised phase II study on neoadjuvant chemotherapy for 'high-risk' adult soft-tissue sarcoma. Eur J Cancer 2001;37(9):1096–103.

20. Callegaro D, Miceli R, Bonvalot S, et al. Development and external validation of two nomograms to predict overall survival and occurrence of distant metastases

in adults after surgical resection of localised soft-tissue sarcomas of the extremities: a retrospective analysis. Lancet Oncol 2016;17(5):671–80.

21. Voss RK, Callegaro D, Chiang YJ, et al. Sarculator is a good model to predict survival in resected extremity and trunk sarcomas in US patients. Ann Surg Oncol 2022.

22. Squires MH, Ethun CG, Donahue EE, et al. Extremity soft tissue sarcoma: a multi-institutional validation of prognostic nomograms. Ann Surg Oncol 2022;29(5): 3291–301.

23. Pasquali S, Pizzamiglio S, Touati N, et al. The impact of chemotherapy on survival of patients with extremity and trunk wall soft tissue sarcoma: revisiting the results of the EORTC-STBSG 62931 randomised trial. Eur J Cancer 2019;109:51–60.

24. Pasquali S, Palmerini E, Quagliuolo V, et al. Neoadjuvant chemotherapy in high-risk soft tissue sarcomas: a Sarculator-based risk stratification analysis of the ISG-STS 1001 randomized trial. Cancer 2022;128(1):85–93.

25. Gerrand CH, Wunder JS, Kandel RA, et al. Classification of positive margins after resection of soft-tissue sarcoma of the limb predicts the risk of local recurrence. J Bone Joint Surg Br 2001;83(8):1149–55.

26. Fourman MS, Ramsey DC, Kleiner J, et al. Temporizing wound VAC dressing until final negative margins are achieved reduces myxofibrosarcoma local recurrence. Ann Surg Oncol 2021;28(13):9171–6.

27. Blaes AH, Lindgren B, Mulrooney DA, et al. Pathologic femur fractures after limb-sparing treatment of soft-tissue sarcomas. J Cancer Surviv 2010;4(4):399–404.

28. Gortzak Y, Lockwood GA, Mahendra A, et al. Prediction of pathologic fracture risk of the femur after combined modality treatment of soft tissue sarcoma of the thigh. Cancer 2010;116(6):1553–9.

29. Folkert MR, Casey DL, Berry SL, et al. Femoral fracture in primary soft-tissue sarcoma of the thigh and groin treated with intensity-modulated radiation therapy: observed versus expected risk. Ann Surg Oncol 2019;26(5):1326–31.

30. Luthringer M, Schultz J, Gala Z, et al. Scalp reconstruction. In: Thaller SR, Panthaki ZJ, editors. Tips and tricks in plastic surgery. Cham (Switzerland): Springer International Publishing; 2022. p. 313–25.

31. Li GZ, Fairweather M, Wang J, et al. Cutaneous radiation-associated breast angiosarcoma: radicality of surgery impacts survival. Ann Surg 2017;265(4): 814–20.

32. Zagars GK, Ballo MT, Pisters PW, et al. Prognostic factors for patients with localized soft-tissue sarcoma treated with conservation surgery and radiation therapy: an analysis of 1225 patients. Cancer 2003;97(10):2530–43.

33. Sabolch A, Feng M, Griffith K, et al. Risk factors for local recurrence and metastasis in soft tissue sarcomas of the extremity. Am J Clin Oncol 2012;35(2):151–7.

34. Braschi EL, Kharod SM, Morris CG, et al. Reirradiation in conservative salvage of recurrent soft-tissue sarcoma: an analysis of treatment efficacy and toxicities. Am J Clin Oncol 2021;44(12):624–8.

35. Guttmann DM, Frick MA, Carmona R, et al. A prospective study of proton reirradiation for recurrent and secondary soft tissue sarcoma. Radiother Oncol 2017; 124(2):271–6.

36. Alamanda VK, Crosby SN, Archer KR, et al. Amputation for extremity soft tissue sarcoma does not increase overall survival: a retrospective cohort study. Eur J Surg Oncol 2012;38(12):1178–83.

37. Neuwirth MG, Song Y, Sinnamon AJ, et al. Isolated limb perfusion and infusion for extremity soft tissue sarcoma: a contemporary systematic review and meta-analysis. Ann Surg Oncol 2017;24(13):3803–10.

38. Aladin H, Jennings A, Hodges M, et al. Major lower limb amputation audit - intro-duction and implementation of a multimodal perioperative pain management guideline. Br J Pain 2018;12(4):230–7.
39. Borghi B, D'Addabbo M, White PF, et al. The use of prolonged peripheral neural blockade after lower extremity amputation: the effect on symptoms associated with phantom limb syndrome. Anesth Analg 2010;111(5):1308–15.
40. Bosanquet DC, Glasbey JC, Stimpson A, et al. Systematic review and meta-analysis of the efficacy of perineural local anaesthetic catheters after major lower limb amputation. Eur J Vasc Endovasc Surg 2015;50(2):241–9.

Radiation Therapy for Soft Tissue Sarcoma

Indications, Timing, Benefits, and Consequences

Kilian E. Salerno, MD

KEYWORDS

• Soft tissue sarcoma • Limb-sparing surgery • Radiation therapy • Local recurrence
• Local control • Retroperitoneal sarcoma

KEY POINTS

- Optimal management of soft tissue sarcoma involves multidisciplinary evaluation before the initiation of treatment and coordination of care between providers from surgical and orthopedic oncology, radiation oncology, and medical and pediatric oncology to determine appropriate treatments for each patient (including the role for radiation therapy and systemic therapies) and the sequence of treatment modalities.
- The role of radiotherapy for localized soft tissue sarcoma in addition to oncologic resection is for an improvement in local control. Indications for use of radiation therapy are based on the assessment of local recurrence risk.
- Collaboration between the treating surgeon and radiation oncologist is essential for the integration of local therapies and includes recurrence risk assessment, defining areas of concern for close or microscopically positive margins, and discussing planned resection, closure techniques, radiation treatment volumes, and concerns regarding potential wound complications.
- For extremity and superficial truncal soft tissue sarcoma, combined-modality local therapy with wide resection and radiotherapy results in high rates of local control and good functional outcomes. Preoperative radiotherapy is associated with less long-term late toxicity and generally preferred over postoperative radiotherapy for most patients.
- For retroperitoneal sarcoma, the role for radiotherapy is controversial. When radiation therapy is used in addition to surgery, preoperative delivery is preferred.

INTRODUCTION

Multidisciplinary care is essential for optimal clinical outcomes for soft tissue sarcoma (STS); the care team should include providers with sarcoma expertise from surgical and orthopedic oncology, radiation oncology, medical and pediatric oncology, pathology, and musculoskeletal radiology.[1–3] The selection and sequencing of therapies

Radiation Oncology Branch, National Cancer Institute, National Institutes of Health, Building 10 CCR, Room B2-3500, Bethesda, MD 20892, USA
E-mail address: kilian.salerno@nih.gov

Surg Clin N Am 102 (2022) 567–582
https://doi.org/10.1016/j.suc.2022.04.001
0039-6109/22/Published by Elsevier Inc.

surgical.theclinics.com

should be discussed before the initiation of treatment. Close collaboration between surgeon and radiation oncologist is necessary for local therapy decision-making.

The primary treatment modality for localized STS is oncologic wide resection and has evolved from radical resection, such as amputation for extremity tumors, to resection with oncologically appropriate margins.[4-6] In patients at an increased risk of local recurrence, radiation therapy (RT) is used in addition to resection to improve local control and for the preservation of function with limb- or organ-sparing approaches.[4-10] Radiotherapy may be delivered preoperatively or postoperatively, definitively for unresectable or oligometastatic disease, and palliatively for symptom management.

This article reviews the role of radiotherapy in the treatment of localized resectable STS with a focus on the management of extremity, truncal, and retroperitoneal sarcoma and addresses indications, timing, benefits, and consequences of RT.

RADIATION THERAPY IN THE TREATMENT OF EXTREMITY AND SUPERFICIAL TRUNCAL SOFT TISSUE SARCOMA

The National Cancer Institute (NCI) I prospective clinical trial established the role for radiotherapy with limb-sparing resection for STS. Patients with high-grade STS were randomized to limb salvage surgery with postoperative RT or amputation. Both arms received chemotherapy. There was no statistical difference in disease-free survival (71% vs 78% p=0.75) or overall survival (83% vs 88% p=0.99) at 5 years between the limb-sparing and the amputation groups, respectively. Four local recurrences occurred in the limb-sparing group. Positive margins were associated with an increased risk of local recurrence (p<0.0001).[4]

The NCI II study further evaluated the role for RT in the setting of limb-sparing resection. Patients with high-grade or low-grade STS were randomized to surgery and postoperative RT or surgery alone. Patients with high-grade disease received adjuvant chemotherapy. Postoperative RT reduced local recurrence without an impact on rates of distant metastasis or overall survival. With long-term follow-up, the local recurrence rate was 1.4% with limb-sparing surgery and RT versus 25% with limb-sparing surgery alone (p=0.0001). The results also suggested that selected patients at a low risk of recurrence could be managed with resection alone.[5,6]

The addition of radiotherapy to resection was also evaluated on a trial of adjuvant brachytherapy (iridium-192 implant) versus no brachytherapy after complete resection of extremity or truncal STS. The addition of RT improved local control with no impact on distant metastases, disease-specific survival, or overall survival. At 5 years, the overall local control was 82% with brachytherapy versus 69% without brachytherapy (p=0.04).[7] The reduction in local recurrence with brachytherapy was seen in patients with high-grade sarcoma; however, unlike the NCI II trial, a local control benefit for low-grade sarcoma was not observed.[5-7]

These trials show that the addition of RT to wide resection improves local control with no adverse impact on overall survival and, for extremity STS, established limb-sparing resection with RT as the standard approach for function preservation, replacing amputation or radical resection for most patients.[4-7]

Indications for Addition of Radiation Therapy to Resection

Use of RT depends on an overall assessment of risk for local recurrence. Risk is based on the complex interplay of patient, tumor, and treatment factors; including the natural history of the histopathologic subtype, anatomic site, tumor grade, size, adjacent critical normal structures, the ability to obtain a negative-margin oncologic resection, and potential consequences of a local recurrence. Previous unplanned excisions or poorly planned biopsies impact recurrence risk and may compromise outcomes.

Radiotherapy is indicated when further improvement in local control beyond that anticipated with wide resection is clinically meaningful, when risk for local recurrence is high, when the consequences of a local recurrence are significant, or when options for management of recurrent disease would be limited.

Factors associated with local recurrence risk

Risk factors and the relative importance of each vary throughout the literature. The most consistent and important prognostic risk factor for local recurrence is margin status.[4,7,11–13] Macroscopic positive margins are associated with significantly high rates of local recurrence.[4,14] Microscopically positive or close margins differ in their risk for recurrence based on whether they are anticipated or planned.[8,14,15] Unanticipated close or positive margins are associated with an increased risk for local recurrence as compared with planned or anticipated close margins proximate to a critical structure including vessel, nerve, or bone.[14,15] In the setting of macroscopic positive margins or unanticipated close or positive margins, the feasibility of re-resection for negative margins and the role for radiotherapy should be discussed.[15–18]

Anatomic location and size of the primary tumor impact the ability to obtain widely negative margins. These variables are important for local recurrence risk but are also prognostic for distant recurrence risk and outcome. Grade is another important risk factor; however, higher grade more accurately predicts the risk for distant metastatic disease and sarcoma-related death.[11,13] Both high-grade and low-grade tumors can have risk for local recurrence.[5,7,8,13]

Given significant differences in natural history, histopathologic subtype is an important factor associated with local recurrence risk. For example, myxofibrosarcoma is highly infiltrative, particularly in subcutaneous tissues, and has a propensity for multiple local recurrences but carries less metastatic risk.[19] Malignant peripheral nerve sheath tumors (MPNST) are also highly infiltrative and associated with not only an increased local recurrence risk but also high metastatic risk.[20] Given the infiltrative spread of these histologies, often with microscopic extension beyond the disease visible on imaging, positive resection margins are not uncommon; therefore, RT is often used to improve local control.[19,20]

Compared with other histopathologic subtypes, myxoid liposarcomas are considered relatively more responsive to RT, significant volume reductions have been seen with preoperative RT, and local control rates are excellent.[21,22] Given this clinical radiosensitivity, the DOREMY study (Dose Reduction of Preoperative Radiotherapy in Myxoid Liposarcoma) evaluated preoperative dose reduction to 3600 cGy. The results of this prospective, single-arm phase II trial suggest dose de-intensification in this setting may provide comparable local control as seen with more standard radiation doses but with less morbidity.[23]

Resection Alone for Soft Tissue Sarcoma

Patients evaluated in studies of STS resection alone often had T1 or low-grade tumors. In selected series, 10-year local control rates of 90% were achieved with function-preserving surgery, higher with margins ≥ 1 cm.[24,25] A nomogram developed to predict local recurrence in patients treated with limb-sparing surgery alone includes age, size, margin status, grade, and histology and can be useful in risk assessment.[13] Surgical wide resection alone is appropriate in selected patients, often those with low-grade disease, small superficial tumors, or small intramuscular tumors for which widely negative margins can be achieved.

Timing of Radiation Therapy When Combined with Wide Resection

In the original studies of resection combined with RT, the RT was delivered postoperatively.[4–7] The National Cancer Institute Canada (NCIC) SR2 trial evaluated the timing of radiotherapy in combination with limb-sparing resection. Patients were randomized to preoperative RT (5000 cGy) versus postoperative RT (6000–6600 cGy). The primary endpoint was major wound healing complications. The study was stopped early when a planned interim analysis found more acute wound healing complications with preoperative RT versus postoperative RT (35% vs 17% p=0.01). Predictors for wound complications with preoperative RT included tumor size (>10 cm) and anatomic site (i.e., lower extremities). Local control was similar with either radiation approach.[9] With longer follow-up, preoperative RT was associated with less late toxicity (i.e., fibrosis, joint stiffness, and edema) as assessed by the Musculoskeletal Tumor Society (MSTS) Rating Scale and the Toronto Extremity Salvage Score (TESS).[26]

Benefits and Consequences of Radiation Therapy

There are no significant differences in local control or survival outcomes between preoperative and postoperative RT, however acute and late toxicities differ.[9,26] Advantages of preoperative RT include potential reduction of seeding and improvement in margin-negative resection rates, clear delineation of tumor "in situ" and areas at risk that can aid in treatment planning, and lower total dose to smaller treatment volumes can reduce late effects (fibrosis, joint stiffness, and edema) with improved functional outcomes. The primary disadvantage of preoperative RT is the increased risk of acute wound complications, particularly in the lower extremity; however, the baseline risk of wound complications following resection alone (without preoperative RT) is not insignificant.[9,10]

An advantage of postoperative RT is a full pathologic evaluation of the resection specimen including surgical margin status, grade, tumor size, and nodal evaluation when applicable. This complete information may obviate RT in select cases. The primary disadvantage of postoperative RT is the delivery of higher doses to larger volumes, leading to increased risk of irreversible late toxicities.[10,26] Postoperative RT may be indicated but delayed or not able to be delivered in the event of prolonged wound healing post resection.

Given the intent for function preservation and reduction of late toxicity, when radiation therapy is indicated based on the anticipated risk for recurrence, preoperative delivery is preferred.[27] Although the risk for acute wound complications is increased with preoperative RT and these complications can cause short-term morbidity and disability, they are usually temporary and reversible, unlike late effects. In some situations, preoperative RT may not be favored, particularly in patients at a significant risk for major wound complications due to multiple additional risk factors for poor healing,and postoperative RT after complete healing following resection may be preferred. The optimal sequence of radiation therapy and resection for each patient should be determined in a multidisciplinary manner, weighing risks for short-term acute wound complications and long-term functional outcomes.

Aspects of Surgical Resection that Impact Radiation Therapy

The treating surgeon and radiation oncologist should discuss the sequence of radiation therapy and resection, planned surgical approach, anticipated closure technique, and tentative plan for management of potential wound complications. Anticipated close or microscopically positive margins due to proximity of the tumor to critical structures are often an indication for use of preoperative RT to improve local

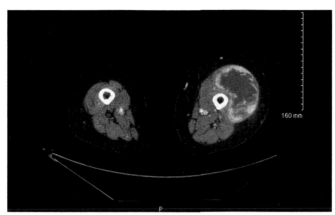

Fig. 1. High-grade undifferentiated pleomorphic sarcoma of the thigh abutting bone with extensive internal necrosis following preoperative radiotherapy. Planning objectives limit dose to the femur, uninvolved soft tissue, and a strip of subcutaneous tissue and skin.

control.[15,28] When noted intraoperatively, the placement of surgical clips to delineate sites or concern for margins is helpful for postoperative target definition. Additionally, plans for resection of the biopsy tract, overlying skin and subcutaneous tissue, periosteal stripping, vascular resection with reconstruction, and the location of drains impact the radiation treatment planning. Periosteal stripping is associated with an increased risk of fracture.[29,30] If periosteal stripping is necessary for tumors directly abutting bone, some sarcoma multidisciplinary teams consider prophylactic intramedullary fixation in select patients at a high risk of fracture, particularly if RT has already been administered or is planned[29,30] (**Fig. 1**). In the setting of an unplanned excision, a similar paradigm for local therapy management can be followed with recurrence risk assessment, role for RT and sequencing with oncologic resection. If salvage wide resection for oncologic margins is not feasible, postoperative RT may be delivered for local control.[27]

Treatment Volumes for External Beam Radiation Therapy

Similar to considerations regarding the extent of resection, in radiation treatment planning there is a balance between margin breadth to reduce local recurrence while sparing the surrounding normal tissues to preserve function. Radiation treatment volumes are defined by sarcoma natural growth patterns longitudinally and radially within a compartment (**Fig. 2**). As subcutaneous tumors are not constrained within a defined compartment, circumferential margins and expansion into underlying muscle are used to define treatment volumes (**Fig. 3**).

Historically, radiation treatment planning margins have been large.[4,5,9] The use of magnetic resonance imaging (MRI) has allowed the refinement of target volumes and a subsequent reduction in radiation treatment margins.[31,32] The use of modern radiation planning and delivery techniques has been investigated to minimize associated toxicities while maintaining local control benefit.[10,33] The RTOG 0630 prospective trial evaluated the use of daily image-guided radiation therapy to further reduce preoperative treatment volumes. High rates of local control were maintained with the use of these reduced expansions, all local recurrences occurred within the treatment fields, and grade ≥ 2 late toxicity at 2 years was 10.5%.[10]

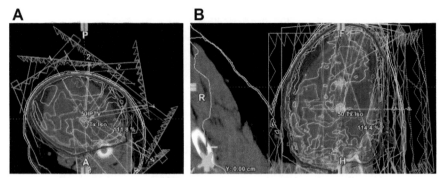

Fig. 2. Prone axial (*A*) and coronal (*B*) images of a preoperative intensity-modulated radiotherapy plan for a posterior thigh sarcoma showing the treatment volume with longitudinal and radial expansions on the tumor (*red contour*). The target volumes are anatomically constrained and do not extend into bone.

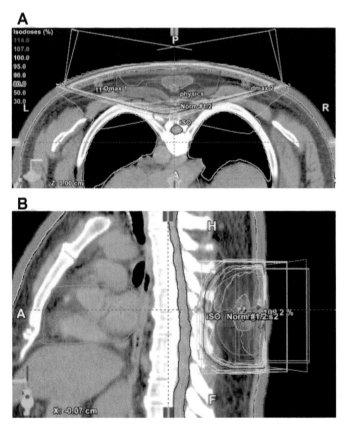

Fig. 3. Prone axial (*A*) and sagittal (*B*) images of a three-dimensional conformal preoperative radiotherapy plan for a subcutaneous high-grade truncal sarcoma complicated by prior unplanned excision with residual disease and seroma. The treatment volume includes circumferential margins on targets and expansion into underlying muscle.

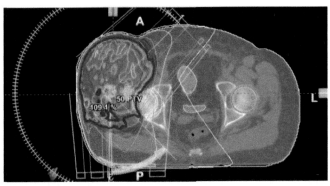

Fig. 4. Preoperative radiotherapy plan for a groin sarcoma using partial volumetric modulated arcs. The treatment volume includes the gross tumor volume with surrounding margin. The expansion does not extend into bone. Planning objectives minimize dose to the femoral head and neck, pelvic organs, and external genitalia. There is no elective nodal irradiation.

Current target definitions for preoperative and postoperative radiation treatment volumes incorporate diagnostic imaging findings (i.e., contrast enhancement and suspicious peritumoral edema seen on MRI). Expansions on gross disease noted on imaging are constrained within anatomic barriers and not extended into uninvolved bone or beyond compartmental fascia for treatment planning. There is no elective nodal irradiation[27,32] (**Fig. 4**).

Ongoing studies are investigating further reductions of dose or treatment volume. The DOREMY study reported initial results of a reduced preoperative RT dose (3600 cGy) for myxoid liposarcoma.[23] The VORTEX trial in the United Kingdom is evaluating whether a smaller postoperative treatment volume can improve limb function while maintaining local control (NCT 00423618). A separate randomized phase III clinical trial of preoperative versus postoperative intensity-modulated RT for extremity and truncal STS is evaluating postoperative dose reduction to 5000 cGy for patients with negative margins (NCT02565498).

Dose and Fractionation for External Beam Radiation Therapy

Preoperative radiation therapy

The majority of clinical trials establishing the role for RT in addition to resection for STS of the extremity and trunk have used conventional fractionation, defined as doses of 180-200 cGy per fraction.[4,5,9,10,33] The current preferred dose for preoperative RT is 5000 cGy in 25 fractions.[27,32] When chemotherapy is given, the total dose and dose per fraction may be reduced to reduce complications.

Postoperative radiation therapy

The total dose for postoperative RT is 6000-6600 cGy as 200 cGy per fraction. Typically, a larger volume encompassing the resection bed, preoperative target with an expansion, incision, and drain sites (when feasible) is treated to 5000 cGy and an additional dose of 1000 cGy (for negative margins) or 1600 cGy (for positive margins) is delivered to a reduced volume, often the tumor bed with an expansion and the area of surgical clips.[27,32] Higher doses may be used for gross residual disease. Courses are often delivered sequentially but may also be treated concurrently using a simultaneous integrated boost.

Hypofractionation
Hypofractionated RT courses deliver larger doses (>200 cGy per fraction) in fewer fractions. Evidence supporting hypofractionated preoperative RT regimens is growing; however, there are no randomized clinical trials comparing shorter courses with conventional fractionation. Most reports suggest acceptable local control rates although studies have used different dose fractionation regimens and timing to resection, limited patient numbers, and variable follow-up and toxicity assessments.[34–38]

Postoperative boost for positive margins or gross disease
Whether a postoperative external beam RT boost in the setting of a positive margin after prior preoperative RT is beneficial for local control is debated, particularly given the prolonged time between completion of preoperative RT and postoperative healing. Boost doses may also be delivered using intraoperative RT and brachytherapy. Some studies found no impact of RT boost on local control whereas others have shown a benefit.[16–18,39] The site of the positive margin, type of margin and whether anticipated or not, and options for subsequent management should be discussed, including the feasibility of re-resection for negative margins. The use of re-resection, postoperative boost, or surveillance should be tailored and often reserved for patients at high risk of recurrence at a well-defined site in whom additional morbidity from RT is expected to be minimal.

Acute and Late Effects of Radiation Therapy

Treatment planning for STS balances the delivery of the prescribed dose to target volumes while minimizing dose to normal adjacent tissues. The relevant normal tissues are dependent on the primary tumor anatomic site. Normal tissue sparing is important for both acute and late effects.

Acute effects of both preoperative or postoperative RT include skin reactions, or dermatitis, which can be more prominent when tumor involves skin or subcutaneous tissues or select anatomic regions with skin folds such as groin, axilla, and gluteal cleft. Dermatitis usually resolves with local skin care and time.

Major wound healing complications are one of the most concerning acute toxicities and attention to planning the dose delivered to skin and subcutaneous tissues can minimize this risk.[40] Radiotherapy planning objectives include sparing a longitudinal strip of uninvolved skin and subcutaneous tissue in the extremity, limiting dose in uninvolved superficial tissues (including the site of planned incision) and skin over areas of frequent trauma, and minimizing dose to joints and weight-bearing bones.[9,10,27,33,40]

In general, late effects are related to both total dose and irradiated volume. In addition to the late effects of fibrosis, joint stiffness, and chronic edema, radiation-associated pathologic fracture is a cause of significant morbidity. Although uncommon, management is challenging with a high risk for delayed union or nonunion.[29,30,41] Fracture risk increases with higher total RT doses, such as delivered with postoperative RT.[6,29,30,41,42] Additional risk factors include bone–dose volume parameters (including circumferential dose), RT technique, extent of periosteal stripping, use of chemotherapy, age, female sex, and tumor size and location.[29,30,41]

For patients with tumors in the upper thigh and pelvis, dose to the external genitalia or perineum and reproductive organs should be minimized; those desiring fertility preservation should be referred for fertility consultation prior to treatment.

Role for Radiotherapy in the Treatment of Retroperitoneal Sarcoma

The primary treatment for a retroperitoneal sarcoma is surgical resection, often with en bloc removal of adjacent viscera while trying to preserve uninvolved organ function.

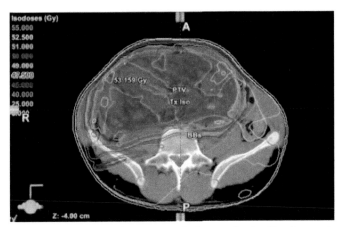

Fig. 5. Preoperative radiotherapy plan to 5000 cGy for a patient with a large retroperitoneal liposarcoma displacing bowel (turquoise contour).

Even with complete macroscopic resection, local recurrence is frequent.[43–46] Histopathologic subtype significantly influences the natural history and risks for local recurrence and hematogenous distant metastatic disease.[43–45] In addition to distant metastases, uncontrolled local disease can result in significant morbidity and mortality. The rationale for RT is for potential local control benefit. However, the use of RT in addition to surgery remains controversial.

The role of RT in addition to resection has limited prospective randomized data; available studies have shown conflicting results and the timing of RT, technique, and modality vary among studies.[8,47–51] The randomized NCI trial compared postoperative external RT to intraoperative electron RT and lower dose postoperative RT.[52] As this study included RT in both arms, it cannot address the role for RT in addition to resection. Two prospective randomized studies evaluating the role for preoperative RT closed prematurely due to poor accrual (RTOG 0124 NCT00017160 and ACOSOG Z9031 NCT00091351).

The EORTC STRASS randomized controlled trial of preoperative RT and surgery versus surgery alone did not show a statistically significant difference in 3-year abdominal recurrence-free survival for the addition of RT to resection. Post-hoc analysis by histopathologic subtype and grade suggested potential improvement in abdominal recurrence-free survival with the addition of preoperative RT for liposarcoma and low-grade sarcoma, without similar benefit for leiomyosarcoma and high-grade sarcoma.[53] A caveat is that the follow-up is relatively short and while the STRASS data do not support routine use of preoperative RT, a combined modality approach may be appropriate in certain circumstances.

The decision regarding whether to add RT to surgery for retroperitoneal sarcoma should be based on multidisciplinary evaluation and assessment of risk for local recurrence in selected patients. When RT is used, preoperative RT is preferred over postoperative RT. Preoperative RT may reduce the risk of tumor seeding and intraperitoneal dissemination at surgery and the tumor being "in situ" often helps to displace adjacent small bowel, thus reducing associated toxicity (**Fig. 5**). Postoperative RT is generally not recommended as the treatment dose exceeds normal tissue tolerance of adjacent organs, the irradiated volume is typically large to encompass the initial extent of disease and surgical bed, and often contains multiple loops of bowel. The dose for preoperative RT is 5000-5040 cGy using conventional

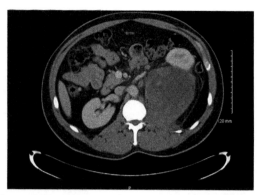

Fig. 6. Contrast-enhanced CT axial image of a retroperitoneal dedifferentiated liposarcoma. Discussion of plan for nephrectomy and evaluation of contralateral renal function are necessary for preoperative radiotherapy planning.

fractionation.[27,53,54] The plan for surgery, especially anticipated ipsilateral nephrectomy or partial hepatic resection, should be reviewed as the extent of resection impacts RT planning and dose constraints to preserve organ function[27,54] (**Fig. 6**). Dose escalation is being studied to provide higher doses to selected volumes at a greater risk of recurrence.[55,56]

OTHER ROLES FOR RADIATION THERAPY IN THE TREATMENT OF SOFT TISSUE SARCOMA
Re-irradiation for Local Recurrence

Management of isolated local recurrence in a previously irradiated field involves surgical resection (when feasible) and, in the setting of prior limb-sparing therapy, may require amputation. In select patients with a localized recurrence amenable to wide resection yet still at significant risk for subsequent recurrence or when radical resection is not possible or declined, re-irradiation may be considered for local control (although with significant risk for wound complications).[57,58] Brachytherapy, advanced planning, or proton RT have been used for re-irradiation to try to minimize normal tissue toxicity.[57–61]

Definitive Radiation Therapy for Unresectable Disease

For patients where limb-sparing resection is not feasible but amputation is unacceptable or for a patient who cannot undergo surgery due to medical comorbidities, definitive RT may be considered for local control albeit with lower rates as compared to resection[62,63] (**Fig. 7**). On one study, local control wass lower with increasing tumor size and higher with greater total dose, however, complications were more frequent with higher dose.[63]

Stereotactic Body Ablative Radiotherapy for Oligometastatic Disease

Stereotactic body ablative radiotherapy (SBAR) or stereotactic body radiation therapy delivers focused large doses of radiation in one or a few fractions to a well-defined tumor volume with ablative intent. Studies show that SBAR is a feasible option for local control of limited pulmonary oligometastatic disease with minimal toxicity[64–67] (**Fig. 8**). This technique has also been used for the treatment of nonpulmonary oligometastases, including liver, spine, soft tissue, and lymph nodes.[68]

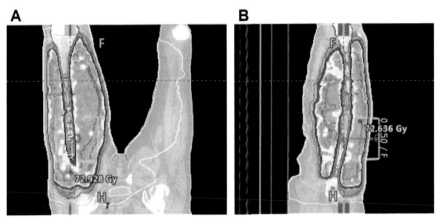

Fig. 7. Coronal (*A*) and sagittal (*B*) images of a definitive radiotherapy plan for high-grade sarcoma involving multiple compartments of the thigh in an elderly patient with medical comorbidities for whom radical resection was not recommended. Note the attempt to spare the length of femur from the full prescription dose.

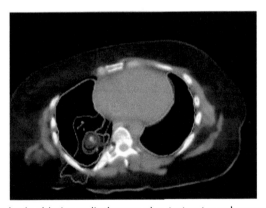

Fig. 8. Stereotactic body ablative radiotherapy plan to treat a pulmonary oligometastasis.

Brachytherapy

The role of brachytherapy in the treatment of STS and technical aspects of use are comprehensively reviewed in the American Brachytherapy Society consensus statement.[61]

SUMMARY

Before the initiation of any sarcoma-directed therapy, a thorough risk assessment should be performed by the multidisciplinary STS team. In patients at an increased risk of local recurrence, RT is indicated, and preoperative delivery of RT is preferred for most patients. When local recurrence risk is low, radiation is not indicated. Oncologic resection alone is appropriate when a high likelihood of local control with widely negative margin resection is anticipated. Some patients initially believed to be at low risk for local recurrence may have unexpected adverse pathologic features following resection (i.e., higher grade disease, larger tumor extent than suspected on preoperative imaging, discontinuous spread, positive margins, or nodal involvement) and are at a high risk of local recurrence. If no prior RT was delivered, postoperative RT is indicated to improve local control. In select patients who received preoperative radiation and have close or positive margins, postoperative boost may be considered. The use of radiation therapy for retroperitoneal sarcoma is controversial. When incorporated into therapy for selected patients at a high risk of local recurrence and morbidity, preoperative delivery of radiation is favored; postoperative RT is not recommended.

CLINICS CARE POINTS

- Seek multidisciplinary input regarding the management before the initiation of sarcoma-directed therapy.

- When determining the role for radiotherapy in the treatment of localized resectable soft tissue sarcoma, assess the risk for local recurrence and consider sites of anticipated close or positive margins before resection.

- Radiation therapy is used to improve local control.

- When radiotherapy is indicated, preoperative delivery is preferred for most patients.

- Discuss with the treating radiation oncologist regarding the sites of concern for margins, risk of local recurrence, plan for resection, and potential for wound healing complications.

- Recognize that the primary tumor often will not "shrink" during preoperative radiotherapy; this is not the intent for use and does not imply that the radiation therapy was ineffective.

- Delineate areas of concern for close of positive margins with surgical clips at the time of resection to facilitate postoperative radiation treatment planning.

DISCLOSURE

No conflicts of interest to disclose.

REFERENCES

1. Blay JY, Honore C, Stoeckle E, et al. Surgery in reference centers improves survival of sarcoma patients: a nationwide study. Ann Oncol 2019;30(8):1407.
2. Blay JY, Soibinet P, Penel N, et al. Improved survival using specialized multidisciplinary board in sarcoma patients. Ann Oncol 2017;28(11):2852–9.
3. Bonvalot S, Gaignard E, Stoeckle E, et al. Survival Benefit of the Surgical Management of Retroperitoneal Sarcoma in a Reference Center: A Nationwide Study of the French Sarcoma Group from the NetSarc Database. Ann Surg Oncol 2019; 26(7):2286–93.
4. Rosenberg SA, Tepper J, Glatstein E, et al. The treatment of soft-tissue sarcomas of the extremities: prospective randomized evaluations of (1) limb-sparing surgery plus radiation therapy compared with amputation and (2) the role of adjuvant chemotherapy. Ann Surg 1982;196(3):305–15.
5. Yang JC, Chang AE, Baker AR, et al. Randomized prospective study of the benefit of adjuvant radiation therapy in the treatment of soft tissue sarcomas of the extremity. J Clin Oncol 1998;16(1):197–203.
6. Beane JD, Yang JC, White D, et al. Efficacy of adjuvant radiation therapy in the treatment of soft tissue sarcoma of the extremity: 20-year follow-up of a randomized prospective trial. Ann Surg Oncol 2014;21(8):2484–9.

7. Pisters PW, Harrison LB, Leung DH, et al. Long-term results of a prospective randomized trial of adjuvant brachytherapy in soft tissue sarcoma. J Clin Oncol 1996;14(3):859–68.
8. Albertsmeier M, Rauch A, Roeder F, et al. External Beam Radiation Therapy for Resectable Soft Tissue Sarcoma: A Systematic Review and Meta-Analysis. Ann Surg Oncol 2018;25(3):754–67.
9. O'Sullivan B, Davis AM, Turcotte R, et al. Preoperative versus postoperative radiotherapy in soft-tissue sarcoma of the limbs: a randomised trial. Lancet 2002;359(9325):2235–41.
10. Wang D, Zhang Q, Eisenberg BL, et al. Significant reduction of late toxicities in patients with extremity sarcoma treated with image-guided radiation therapy to a reduced target volume: results of Radiation Therapy Oncology Group RTOG-0630 Trial. J Clin Oncol 2015;33(20):2231–8.
11. Zagars GK, Ballo MT, Pisters PW, et al. Prognostic factors for patients with localized soft-tissue sarcoma treated with conservation surgery and radiation therapy: an analysis of 1225 patients. Cancer 2003;97(10):2530–43.
12. Pisters PW, Leung DH, Woodruff J, et al. Analysis of prognostic factors in 1,041 patients with localized soft tissue sarcomas of the extremities. J Clin Oncol 1996;14(5):1679–89.
13. Cahlon O, Brannon MF, Jia X, et al. A postoperative nomogram for local recurrence risk in extremity soft tissue sarcomas after limb-sparing surgery without adjuvant radiation. Ann Surg 2012;255(2):343–7.
14. Gundle KR, Kafchinski L, Gupta S, et al. Analysis of Margin Classification Systems for Assessing the Risk of Local Recurrence After Soft Tissue Sarcoma Resection. J Clin Oncol 2018;36(7):704–9.
15. O'Donnell PW, Griffin AM, Eward WC, et al. The effect of the setting of a positive surgical margin in soft tissue sarcoma. Cancer 2014;120(18):2866–75.
16. Delaney TF, Kepka L, Goldberg SI, et al. Radiation therapy for control of soft-tissue sarcomas resected with positive margins. Int J Radiat Oncol Biol Phys 2007;67(5):1460–9.
17. Al Yami A, Griffin AM, Ferguson PC, et al. Positive surgical margins in soft tissue sarcoma treated with preoperative radiation: is a postoperative boost necessary? Int J Radiat Oncol Biol Phys 2010;77(4):1191–7.
18. Pan E, Goldberg SI, Chen YL, et al. Role of post-operative radiation boost for soft tissue sarcomas with positive margins following pre-operative radiation and surgery. J Surg Oncol 2014;110(7):817–22.
19. Boughzala-Bennadji R, Stoeckle E, Le Péchoux C, et al. Localized myxofibrosarcomas: roles of surgical margins and adjuvant radiation therapy. Int J Radiat Oncol Biol Phys 2018;102(2):399–406.
20. Martin E, Coert JH, Flucke UE, et al. A nationwide cohort study on treatment and survival in patients with malignant peripheral nerve sheath tumours. Eur J Cancer 2020;124:77–87.
21. Chung PW, Deheshi BM, Ferguson PC, et al. Radiosensitivity translates into excellent local control in extremity myxoid liposarcoma: a comparison with other soft tissue sarcomas. Cancer 2009;115(14):3254–61.
22. Guadagnolo BA, Zagars GK, Ballo MT, et al. Excellent local control rates and distinctive patterns of failure in myxoid liposarcoma treated with conservation surgery and radiotherapy. Int J Radiat Oncol Biol Phys 2008;70(3):760–5.
23. Lansu J, Bovée JVMG, Braam P, et al. Dose Reduction of preoperative radiotherapy in myxoid liposarcoma: a nonrandomized controlled trial. JAMA Oncol 2021;7(1):e205865.

24. Pisters PW, Pollock RE, Lewis VO, et al. Long-term results of prospective trial of surgery alone with selective use of radiation for patients with T1 extremity and trunk soft tissue sarcomas. Ann Surg 2007;246(4):675–81 [discussion: 681–682].
25. Baldini EH, Goldberg J, Jenner C, et al. Long-term outcomes after function-sparing surgery without radiotherapy for soft tissue sarcoma of the extremities and trunk. J Clin Oncol 1999;17(10):3252–9.
26. Davis A, O'Sullivan B, Turcotte R, et al. Late radiation morbidity following randomization to preoperative versus postoperative radiotherapy in extremity soft tissue sarcoma. Radiother Oncol 2005;75(1):48–53.
27. Salerno KE, Alektiar KM, Baldini EH, et al. Radiation therapy for treatment of soft tissue sarcoma in adults: executive summary of an ASTRO Clinical Practice Guideline. Pract Radiat Oncol 2021;11(5):339–51.
28. Shelby RD, Suarez-Kelly LP, Yu PY, et al. Neoadjuvant radiation improves margin-negative resection rates in extremity sarcoma but not survival. J Surg Oncol 2020; 121:1249–58.
29. Bishop AJ, Zagars GK, Allen PK, et al. Treatment-related fractures after combined modality therapy for soft tissue sarcomas of the proximal lower extremity: Can the risk be mitigated? Pract Radiat Oncol 2016;6(3):194–200.
30. Folkert MR, Casey DL, Berry SL, et al. Femoral fracture in primary soft-tissue sarcoma of the thigh and groin treated with intensity-modulated radiation therapy: observed versus expected risk. Ann Surg Oncol 2019;26(5):1326–31.
31. White LM, Wunder JS, Bell RS, et al. Histologic assessment of peritumoral edema in soft tissue sarcoma. Int J Radiat Oncol Biol Phys 2005;61(5):1439–45.
32. Haas RL, Delaney TF, O'Sullivan B, et al. Radiotherapy for management of extremity soft tissue sarcomas: why, when, and where? Int J Radiat Oncol Biol Phys 2012;84(3):572–80.
33. O'Sullivan B, Griffin AM, Dickie CI, et al. Phase 2 study of preoperative image-guided intensity-modulated radiation therapy to reduce wound and combined modality morbidities in lower extremity soft tissue sarcoma. Cancer 2013; 119(10):1878–84.
34. Kalbasi A, Kamrava M, Chu FI, et al. A Phase II Trial of 5-day neoadjuvant radiotherapy for patients with high-risk primary soft tissue sarcoma. Clin Cancer Res 2020;26:1829–36.
35. Koseła-Paterczyk H, Spałek M, Borkowska A, et al. Hypofractionated radiotherapy in locally advanced myxoid liposarcomas of extremities or trunk wall: results of a single-arm prospective clinical trial. J Clin Med 2020;9(8):2471.
36. Kosela-Paterczyk H, Szacht M, Morysinski T, et al. Preoperative hypofractionated radiotherapy in the treatment of localized soft tissue sarcomas. Eur J Surg Oncol 2014;40(12):1641–7.
37. Pennington JD, Eilber FC, Eilber FR, et al. Long-term Outcomes With Ifosfamide-based Hypofractionated Preoperative Chemoradiotherapy for Extremity Soft Tissue Sarcomas. Am J Clin Oncol 2018;41(12):1154–61.
38. Kubicek GJ, LaCouture T, Kaden M, et al. Preoperative Radiosurgery for Soft Tissue Sarcoma. Am J Clin Oncol 2018;41(1):86–9.
39. Wells S, Ager B, Hitchcock YJ, et al. The radiation dose-response of non-retroperitoneal soft tissue sarcoma with positive margins: an NCDB analysis. J Surg Oncol 2019;120:1476–85.
40. Baldini EH, Lapidus MR, Wang Q, et al. Predictors for major wound complications following preoperative radiotherapy and surgery for soft-tissue sarcoma of the extremities and trunk: importance of tumor proximity to skin surface. Ann Surg Oncol 2013;20(5):1494–9.

41. Dickie CI, Parent AL, Griffin AM, et al. Bone fractures following external beam radiotherapy and limb-preservation surgery for lower extremity soft tissue sarcoma: relationship to irradiated bone length, volume, tumor location and dose. Int J Radiat Oncol Biol Phys 2009;75(4):1119–24.

42. Pak D, Vineberg KA, Griffith KA, et al. Dose–effect relationships for femoral fractures after multimodality limb-sparing therapy of soft-tissue sarcomas of the proximal lower extremity. Int J Radiat Oncol Biol Phys 2012;83(4):1257–63.

43. Gronchi A, Strauss DC, Miceli R, et al. Variability in patterns of recurrence after resection of primary retroperitoneal sarcoma (RPS): a report on 1007 patients from the multi-institutional collaborative rps working group. Ann Surg 2016; 263(5):1002–9.

44. Tan MC, Brennan MF, Kuk D, et al. Histology-based classification predicts pattern of recurrence and improves risk stratification in primary retroperitoneal sarcoma. Ann Surg 2016;263(3):593–600.

45. Gronchi A, Lo Vullo S, Fiore M, et al. Aggressive surgical policies in a retrospectively reviewed single-institution case series of retroperitoneal soft tissue sarcoma patients. J Clin Oncol 2009;27(1):24–30.

46. Bonvalot S, Rivoire M, Castaing M, et al. Primary retroperitoneal sarcomas: a multivariate analysis of surgical factors associated with local control. J Clin Oncol 2009;27(1):31–7.

47. Pawlik TM, Pisters PW, Mikula L, et al. Long-term results of two prospective trials of preoperative external beam radiotherapy for localized intermediate- or high-grade retroperitoneal soft tissue sarcoma. Ann Surg Oncol 2006;13(4):508–17.

48. Kelly KJ, Yoon SS, Kuk D, et al. Comparison of perioperative radiation therapy and surgery versus surgery alone in 204 patients with primary retroperitoneal sarcoma: a retrospective 2-institution study. Ann Surg 2015;262(1):156–62.

49. Bishop AJ, Zagars GK, Torres KE, et al. Combined modality management of retroperitoneal sarcomas: a single-institution series of 121 patients. Int J Radiat Oncol Biol Phys 2015;93(1):158–65.

50. Nussbaum DP, Speicher PJ, Gulack BC, et al. Long-term oncologic outcomes after neoadjuvant radiation therapy for retroperitoneal sarcomas. Ann Surg 2015; 262(1):163–70.

51. Chouliaras K, Senehi R, Ethun CG, et al. Role of radiation therapy for retroperitoneal sarcomas: An eight-institution study from the US Sarcoma Collaborative. J Surg Oncol 2019;120(7):1227–34.

52. Sindelar WF, Kinsella TJ, Chen PW, et al. Intraoperative radiotherapy in retroperitoneal sarcomas. Final results of a prospective, randomized, clinical trial. Arch Surg 1993;128(4):402–10.

53. Bonvalot S, Gronchi A, Le Péchoux C, et al. Preoperative radiotherapy plus surgery versus surgery alone for patients with primary retroperitoneal sarcoma (EORTC-62092: STRASS): a multicentre, open-label, randomised, phase 3 trial. Lancet Oncol 2020;21(10):1366–77.

54. Baldini EH, Wang D, Haas RL, et al. Treatment guidelines for preoperative radiation therapy for retroperitoneal sarcoma: preliminary consensus of an international expert panel. Int J Radiat Oncol Biol Phys 2015;92(3):602–12.

55. McBride SM, Raut CP, Lapidus M, et al. Locoregional recurrence after preoperative radiation therapy for retroperitoneal sarcoma: adverse impact of multifocal disease and potential implications of dose escalation. Ann Surg Oncol 2013; 20(7):2140–7.

56. DeLaney TF, Chen YL, Baldini EH, et al. Phase 1 trial of preoperative image guided intensity modulated proton radiation therapy with simultaneously

integrated boost to the high risk margin for retroperitoneal sarcomas. Adv Radiat Oncol 2017;2(1):85–93.

57. Guttmann DM, Frick MA, Carmona R, et al. A prospective study of proton reirradiation for recurrent and secondary soft tissue sarcoma. Radiother Oncol 2017; 124(2):271–6.

58. Indelicato DJ, Meadows K, Gibbs CP Jr, et al. Effectiveness and morbidity associated with reirradiation in conservative salvage management of recurrent soft-tissue sarcoma. Int J Radiat Oncol Biol Phys 2009;73(1):267–72.

59. Torres MA, Ballo MT, Butler CE, et al. Management of locally recurrent soft-tissue sarcoma after prior surgery and radiation therapy. Int J Radiat Oncol Biol Phys 2007;67(4):1124–9.

60. Catton C, Davis A, Bell R, et al. Soft tissue sarcoma of the extremity. Limb salvage after failure of combined conservative therapy. Radiother Oncol 1996;41(3): 209–14.

61. Naghavi AO, Fernandez DC, Mesko N, et al. American Brachytherapy Society consensus statement for soft tissue sarcoma brachytherapy. Brachytherapy 2017;16(3):466–89.

62. Tepper JE, Suit HD. Radiation therapy alone for sarcoma of soft tissue. Cancer 1985;56(3):475–9.

63. Kepka L, DeLaney TF, Suit HD, et al. Results of radiation therapy for unresected soft-tissue sarcomas. Int J Radiat Oncol Biol Phys 2005;63(3):852–9.

64. Baumann BC, Bernstein KA, DeLaney TF, et al. Multi-institutional analysis of stereotactic body radiotherapy for sarcoma pulmonary metastases: High rates of local control with favorable toxicity. J Surg Oncol 2020;122(5):877–83.

65. Baumann BC, Nagda SN, Kolker JD, et al. Efficacy and safety of stereotactic body radiation therapy for the treatment of pulmonary metastases from sarcoma: a potential alternative to resection. J Surg Oncol 2016;114(1):65–9.

66. Navarria P, Ascolese AM, Cozzi L, et al. Stereotactic body radiation therapy for lung metastases from soft tissue sarcoma. Eur J Cancer 2015;51:668–74.

67. Dhakal S, Corbin KS, Milano MT, et al. Stereotactic body radiotherapy for pulmonary metastases from soft-tissue sarcomas: excellent local lesion control and improved patient survival. Int J Radiat Oncol Biol Phys 2012;82(2):940–5.

68. Folkert MR, Bilsky MH, Tom AK, et al. Outcomes and toxicity for hypofractionated and single-fraction image-guided stereotactic radiosurgery for sarcomas metastasizing to the spine. Int J Radiat Oncol Biol Phys 2014;88:1085–91.

Plastic Surgery Reconstruction of Sarcoma Resection Defects: Form and Function

Zachary E. Stiles, DO, MS[a], Robert F. Lohman, MD, MBA[b],
Gary N. Mann, MD[a,c],*

KEYWORDS

• Sarcoma • Reconstruction • Flap • Pedicle flap • Free flap • Limb salvage

KEY POINTS

• Multimodality therapy has significantly increased rates of limb-sparing resection for sarcoma, often necessitating reconstruction of resection defects.
• Following adequate oncologic resection, reconstruction should focus on preserving functional and cosmetic outcomes while minimizing postoperative morbidity.
• The simplest available reconstructive option should be considered first, but a more complex reconstruction may be required.

INTRODUCTION

Sarcomas are a heterogeneous group of malignancies arising from bone and soft tissue that currently represent 6% to 15% and less than 1% of all malignancies in the pediatric and adult populations, respectively.[1-3] Surgical wide resection is the mainstay of treatment. Given the need for wide resection to obtain negative margins, primary closure of the resection defect often may not be possible. This article includes a discussion of considerations for closure of these frequently complex wounds and is relevant for both the resecting and the reconstructing surgeon.

Historical Perspective

Radical resection was once the only possible means of treatment of soft tissue sarcomas. Historically, amputation had been the standard of care for extremity sarcomas and, even just several decades ago, was performed in up to 50% of cases.[4-6] The

[a] Department of Surgical Oncology, Roswell Park Comprehensive Cancer Center, 128 Carlton Street, 6th Floor, Buffalo, NY, 14263, USA; [b] Department of Plastic and Reconstructive Surgery, Roswell Park Comprehensive Cancer Center, 128 Carlton Street, 7th Floor, Buffalo, NY, 14263, USA; [c] Department of Surgical Oncology, Roswell Park Comprehensive Cancer Center, 128 Carlton Street, 6th Floor, Buffalo, NY 14263, USA
* Corresponding author.
E-mail address: gary.mann@roswellpark.org

Surg Clin N Am 102 (2022) 583–599
https://doi.org/10.1016/j.suc.2022.04.008
0039-6109/22/© 2022 Elsevier Inc. All rights reserved.
surgical.theclinics.com

utilization of appropriate systemic chemotherapy along with more effective radiation therapy has led to not only better disease-specific outcomes, but also greater rates of limb salvage operations for extremity sarcomas.[7–12] With more recent series citing major amputation rates of only 6%,[13] clearly reconstructive options need to be considered to optimize postoperative functional and esthetic outcomes.

Goals of Resection and Reconstruction

There are 3 central themes that should be considered when planning a surgical approach and reconstruction:

1. Wide resection should be focused on achieving oncologically appropriate negative margins.
2. Reconstruction should strive to preserve function and, ideally, an acceptable esthetic result.
3. Postoperative morbidity should be minimal for both the resection and reconstruction.[14–16]

An appropriate oncologic operation should supersede all reconstructive concerns. After an oncologically appropriate resection has been performed, reconstruction can proceed. If there are concerns about possible positive margins, reconstruction may need to be delayed until full pathologic assessment can be performed. Many times, there will be multiple acceptable reconstructive options available to the plastic surgeon. Ultimately, each case should be individualized and take into consideration the cost and institutional resources in addition to anatomic factors and the patient's functional status.

Multidisciplinary Approach

Sarcoma resection and the subsequent reconstruction can be a complex endeavor, and, at a minimum, requires input from a surgical or orthopedic oncologist and a plastic surgeon. However, advice from other specialists, including radiation and medical oncologists, is often helpful. The complexity of the reconstruction may also be increased with large tumors, sensitive or difficult anatomic locations, and in cases of previous operations or recurrent disease. Given these intricacies, preoperative planning is a prerequisite. The reconstructing plastic surgeon should be involved when planning the resection so as not to limit reconstructive options. It is important to maintain access to adjacent healthy soft tissue, which may serve as a suitable donor for reconstruction. Recipient vessels for possible vascular grafts or free tissue transfers should also be considered and kept in mind when performing the resection.[17–19] At times, it may be necessary to involve an orthopedic surgeon for the reconstruction. Bony fixation may be required before soft tissue coverage. Less often, vascularized bone transfer may be necessary to span significant gaps in the bone after resection.[18,20,21]

As many cases of limb salvage surgery for sarcoma will involve radiation therapy, it is imperative to involve radiation oncologists early during treatment planning in cases in which external beam radiation will be delivered. Previous radiation therapy or plans for radiation in the future can both potentially influence the choice of reconstruction. Preoperative doses of radiation are usually lower than when radiation is used postresection. However, consensus guidelines still recommend treatment margins 3 cm beyond the tumor grossly, both proximally and distally, and a 1.5-cm radial treatment margin.[22] Given the potential large size of these radiation fields and the fact that a primarily closed wound in an irradiated bed is at higher risk for postoperative complications, additional reconstructive options should be considered. Wound healing time and the risk of wound complications should be considered when selecting a reconstructive option in cases in which postoperative radiation is planned. A delay in the initiation of adjuvant radiotherapy can occur in cases with acute wound complications.[23] Scars and drain sites should also be contemplated because these need to be included in the treatment field when postoperative radiation is used.[24]

In many cases, the success of the reconstructive plan also depends on the contribution of supportive care services. Physical and occupational therapy should be involved either before surgery ("prehab") or early in the postoperative course to improve functional outcomes.[25] Many patients will require some type of postoperative rehabilitation, and rehabilitation practitioners should be involved in treatment planning. Issues related to treatment such as muscle loss, extremity edema, soft tissue fibrosis, contracture formation, and neuropraxia can be addressed.[26] These concerns can be seen in both the acute and long-term phases of recovery. Therefore, continued reassessment and patient education regarding their rehabilitation are crucial to maintenance of lasting function.[27]

DISCUSSION
General Considerations

In general, the simplest and most effective closure or reconstruction technique should be considered first for every case. Reconstructing methods of increasing complexity can then be applied as each case dictates. This concept, known as the "reconstructive ladder," is a central principle in the field of plastic and reconstructive surgery. Primary closure and healing by secondary intention make up the lower rungs of the ladder, whereas distant and free flaps are on the highest rungs. Updated iterations of the reconstructive ladder have also included newer closure methods and tools such as dermal matrices and negative pressure wound therapy (NPWT) **(Fig. 1)**.[28] It may not always be practical to progress up the ladder when choosing a closure technique. Rather, it may be more appropriate to skip over the lower rungs of the ladder and go directly to one of the more complex techniques when it results in a more efficient and definitive result. This framework, known as the reconstructive elevator, allows the reconstructing surgeon to customize the approach to each case and choose the best option for each patient.[29]

Preoperative Planning

The patient should meet with both the surgical/orthopedic oncologist and reconstructive surgeon preoperatively. As part of the preoperative evaluation, comorbidities including cardiac and pulmonary disease should be optimized. Nutritional deficiencies should be recognized, and patients should be counseled on dietary or caloric supplementation if necessary. Smoking and nicotine cessation for at least 6 to 8 weeks preoperatively should be stressed. For diabetics, glycemic control should be maintained in the perioperative period because hyperglycemia is a known risk factor for surgical site infection (SSI) and wound dehiscence.[30] In some patients, referral to physical and occupation therapy may be made preoperatively for prehabilitation and educational preparation for the postoperative period.

Anatomic Considerations

Truncal sarcomas
Chest wall. Chest wall resections primarily involve soft tissues but, in some instances, will include deeper structures such as ribs, costal cartilage, or intercostal muscles. Reconstruction of the chest wall should focus on: (1) reestablishing structural integrity to ensure proper mobility and pulmonary function, (2) providing an airtight closure if

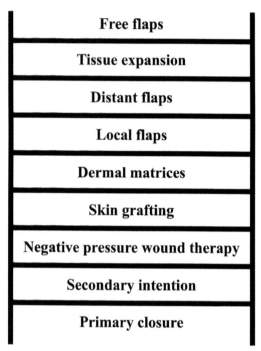

| Free flaps |
| Tissue expansion |
| Distant flaps |
| Local flaps |
| Dermal matrices |
| Skin grafting |
| Negative pressure wound therapy |
| Secondary intention |
| Primary closure |

Fig. 1. Reconstructive ladder ranging from simple closure methods at the bottom to more complex techniques at the top.

the pleural cavity is violated during resection, and (3) restoring soft tissue coverage, which ensures an acceptable cosmetic result. In general, resection defects following sternectomy or resection of up to 4 ribs can undergo soft tissue reconstruction alone.[31–33] There is concern for development of flail chest with larger defects, and reconstruction in these cases typically involves mesh. Multiple options for mesh exist including both nonrigid (polytetrafluoroethylene, polypropylene, and various biologic materials) and rigid constructs (vicryl or polypropylene mesh with methyl methacrylate) (**Fig. 2**).[34–36] Resorbable or metal plates can also be used for larger defects. Morbidity following chest wall reconstruction correlates to the size of the resection defect and may include pneumonia, respiratory failure, and prolonged air leak.[37] Myocutaneous flaps are typically used for soft tissue coverage of larger defects because they help obliterate dead space and cover synthetic material when mesh is used.[36] Among flaps, the pedicled latissimus dorsi (LD) flap has become the workhorse for chest wall coverage.[35] Other options include the vertical rectus abdominis myocutaneous (VRAM) flap, serratus anterior muscle flap, or trapezius flap.[36] Less commonly, the omentum may also be used as a reconstruction option, especially when infection is a concern or more common pedicle flaps are not an option.[38]

Abdominal wall. The extent of abdominal wall reconstruction varies significantly depending on the defect size and depth, which may be partially attributed to the type of tumor resected. Desmoid tumors and soft tissue sarcomas tend to be close to or involve the musculofascial planes, whereas other tumors such as dermatofibrosarcoma protuberans are typically more superficial and do not involve the fascial layers.[39,40] It is important to identify cases preoperatively that might involve gastrointestinal tract violation. These wounds will be at greater risk for SSI and hernia

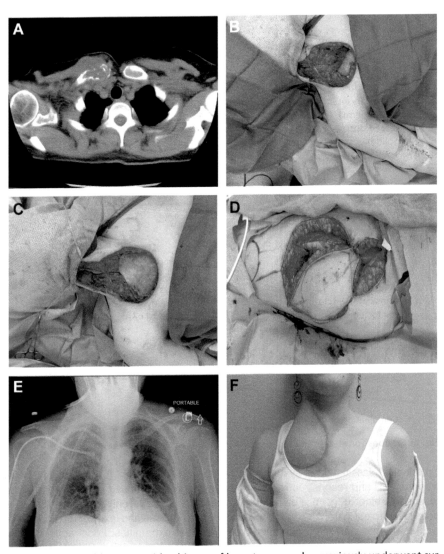

Fig. 2. A 39-year-old woman with a history of breast cancer who previously underwent surgical resection and external beam radiation therapy. (A) She later developed a radiation-associated high-grade osteosarcoma of the right clavicular head. (B) Following wide excision of the tumor, including the medial aspect of the clavicle, a large resection defect remained. The exposed apex of the lung can be seen in the inferior aspect of the wound. (C) Ovine-derived bioprosthetic mesh (Ovitex [Aroa Biosurgery, New Zealand]) was sutured in place over the exposed lung for thoracic cavity reconstruction. (D) An ALT flap is prepared for reconstruction of the defect with 2 perforators marked in the long axis of the flap. (E) A frontal chest radiograph obtained postoperatively with a thoracostomy tube in place shows good expansion of the right lung with no evidence of significant pneumothorax or effusion. (F) Appearance of the flap after healing.

formation; this will influence reconstructive choices, including the use of synthetic mesh.[41] Ultimately, reconstruction should focus on providing a durable repair that minimizes the risk of future abdominal wall weakness or hernia formation while providing soft tissue coverage over any fascial repair.

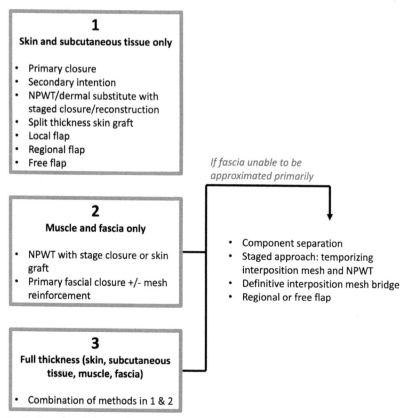

Fig. 3. Options for abdominal reconstruction based on depth of wound.

Multiple classification systems have been developed for abdominal wall wounds,[42,43] and reconstructive options can be grouped based on the depth of the resection defect (**Fig. 3**). For defects involving soft tissue only, primary closure is possible in many instances due to the abundance of tissue and laxity of the abdominal wall compared with more constricted areas in the extremities. Local advancement flaps can be used to provide a tension-free closure of an incision. Skin grafting may also be used for superficial wounds when the skin edges cannot be fully approximated. At times, a simpler method such as primary closure or skin grafting may be preferable for tumors such as DFSP that have a higher recurrence rate.[40] For wounds involving the fascia, component separation is often necessary, but the extent of component separation is variable based on the size of the fascial defect. Mesh reinforcement is superior to suture repair alone and reduces the risk of future hernia recurrence.[44] Synthetic, biologic, and hybrid meshes are available. In cases in which the fascia cannot be reapproximated primarily, mesh can be used in an interposition fashion, although this should be avoided, if possible, because this technique is associated with the greatest risk of hernia and/or abdominal wall weakness.[42,45] Local or pedicled flaps such as a pedicled rectus femoris or anterolateral thigh (ALT) flap can be used if the soft tissue is unable to be closed over a mesh repair (**Figs. 4–6**). Propeller perforator flaps may also be used for soft tissue reconstruction of the trunk.[46,47] For larger full-thickness defects where a pedicled flap is not an option, free tissue transfer such as a free ALT flap can be used.[48–50]

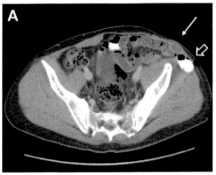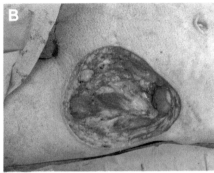

Fig. 4. A 51-year-old man who had previously undergone multiple resections of a recurrent high-grade malignant fibrous histiocytoma was noted to have an enlarging palpable mass near the area of his previous resections on the left lower abdominal wall. He had also previously received radiation therapy to the area. (*A*) Preoperative computed tomography demonstrates a 3-cm peripherally enhancing mass with central low density corresponding to the palpable mass (*solid white arrow*). Core biopsies were performed and showed recurrent high-grade undifferentiated pleomorphic sarcoma. Herniation of bowel, likely as a result of previous resections in the area, can be seen lateral to the iliac spine (*empty white arrow*). (*B*) The patient underwent wide resection of the recurrent left lower anterior abdominal wall sarcoma with en bloc full-thickness resection of the abdominal wall including the inguinal ligament and previously placed mesh. Exposed bowel can be seen at the cephalad aspect of the wound.

Extremity sarcomas
Upper extremity. For the extremities, the extent of reconstruction and potential options will vary significantly depending on the location of the resection defect. Near the shoulder, more soft tissue is available for local flaps and several robust regional flaps (pectoralis, latissimus, scapular, and so on) are available. Distal to the elbow, there are fewer options for local flaps. In the forearm, most muscles available for transfer also contribute to motion of the hand and wrist and closure of the donor sites can be difficult. Tumor resection frequently involves sacrifice of functional muscle, tendon or nerves. Therefore, reconstruction of multiple tissue types is more likely to be required following resection of upper extremity sarcomas.[51]

Single-stage reconstruction is preferred, including nerve and tendon transfers, soft tissue coverage, and rigid bone grafting/fixation as needed. Compared with truncal sarcomas, tumors involving the extremities are more likely to require bone and joint reconstruction, which requires advanced planning and almost always involves help from an orthopedic surgeon. Segmental bony allografts or autografts may be required, particularly for longer or periarticular gaps. If a vascularized bone graft is needed, the free fibula graft with or without a skin paddle is most often used.[52,53] Fixation should be robust enough to tolerate immediate or early weight-bearing. If joint replacement or fusion is required, the associated hardware must be sealed under a well-perfused and durable layer of soft tissue.

Proximally, the LD myocutaneous flap can be used around the shoulder as well as the anterior and posterior surfaces of the upper arm.[54,55] There are limited soft tissue flaps available for use in the hand and forearm. Skin grafting is an option but alone does not provide an adequate gliding surface over joints and other mobile structures. As a result, skin grafts can be fragile and associated with other issues such as contracture and hypersensitivity. In many circumstances, these risks can be mitigated by staged application of skin grafts over a dermal substitute. The most common method of soft tissue

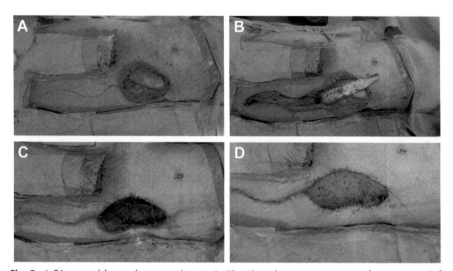

Fig. 5. A 51-year-old man (same patient as in **Fig. 4**) underwent resection of a recurrent left lower anterior abdominal wall sarcoma with en bloc full-thickness resection of the abdominal wall including the inguinal ligament. Reconstruction was performed with a pedicled rectus femoris flap and split-thickness skin grafting. (A) Bioprosthetic mesh was used to restore the abdominal wall and inguinal ligament. The donor site for the rectus femoris flap was marked. (B) The flap was harvested and rotated over the defect to cover the mesh. The origin of the extensor tendon, visible in this image, was subsequently excised to facilitate adherence of a skin graft. (C) The flap was sutured in place and the donor site was closed primarily. (D) A split-thickness skin graft was applied over the muscle flap.

coverage for wounds between the hand and elbow is the radial forearm flap.[56] However, these operations can be quite long with a tourniquet in place and often involve extensive rehabilitation after surgery when the patient may be preoccupied with adjuvant therapy. For these reasons, one option is to consider performing tendon and nerve transfer surgery while the patient is undergoing neoadjuvant chemotherapy/radiation, before the actual tumor resection. This approach can greatly simplify care after surgery and minimizes the functional deficit immediately after tumor resection. These long-term functional aspects of reconstruction should be kept in mind, especially for areas such as the hand that are integral to day-to-day personal and occupational function.[57–59] Occupational and physical therapists, prosthetics specialists, rehabilitation providers, and occasionally pain medicine physicians may need to be involved to maximize function after upper extremity surgery. Given the lack of other suitable pedicled flaps, the next choice for reconstruction for both the upper and lower arms would be free tissue transfer, often with either ALT or LD free flaps.[19,50]

Lower extremity. The thigh is the most common location of extremity soft tissue sarcomas, likely attributable to its greater tissue mass.[1] Given the greater amounts of soft tissue in the thigh, primary closure or local rotational flaps may be possible reconstructive options. However, much like the upper extremity, reconstructive options become limited more distally on the lower extremity. Again, many of the same concerns exist, such as the need to cover neurovascular structures or the difficulty in addressing coverage of the joints. From a functional and recovery standpoint, it is also important to consider the short- and long-term effects reconstruction has on ambulation and the patient's weight-bearing status.[60]

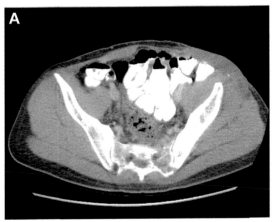
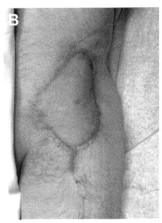

Fig. 6. Following reconstruction with a rectus femoris flap and split-thickness skin graft (same patient as in **Fig. 5**), the 51-year-old man was seen in follow-up. (*A*) Follow-up computed tomography, 6 months following reconstruction. Expected postsurgical soft tissue changes can be seen with visualization of the in situ rectus femoris flap. There is no evidence of bowel herniation. (*B*) Healed appearance of the flap and skin graft several months following surgery.

Local advancement and rotational flaps are both useful when primary closure is not possible. Among these, V-Y advancement and keystone perforator flaps are versatile options for coverage of small- to medium-sized soft tissue defects.[61–63] However, the complication rate for these flaps can be high when they are used to close a wound in previously irradiated tissue. More robust coverage is typically required for wounds with larger defects, exposed neurovascular structures, or when preoperative radiation has been used. For the proximal thigh, pedicled VRAM flaps are the most reliable option and provide abundant healthy tissue.[64–66] Pedicled ALT flaps are an alternative option to manage wounds around the hip, pelvis, and lower abdomen.[67] Regional skin flaps are rarely required for closure of wounds in the central portion of the thigh. The exception to this rule is for prophylactic coverage of an irradiated femur that has been stripped of its periosteum. In this setting, covering the femur with a well-perfused layer of tissue may reduce the risk of pathologic fracture. More distally, propeller flaps can be used.[68] The most common pedicled options are the gastrocnemius or reverse ALT.[69] The soleus is classically used for the middle third of the leg, and the reverse sural flap will reach to the foot and ankle.[14,70] Similar to the upper extremity, local and regional tissue transfer options become more limited lower on the leg. Small wounds of the leg can be covered with anterior tibialis muscle, variations of the sural flap, or local tissue rearrangement. However, larger defects of the distal third of the leg, ankle, or foot often require free tissue transfer.[18,50,71–73] Thin pliable flaps, such as the radial forearm or ALT skin flap, are preferred. Bulky muscle or myocutaneous flaps should be avoided, if possible; otherwise it may be difficult for the patient to use normal footwear.

Special Considerations

Unusual anatomic locations

Hand. Sarcomas of the hand are uncommon but present challenges regarding reconstruction when they do occur. Finger and ray amputations may be required for sarcoma of the digits, but transradial amputation is rarely necessary. Given the density of structures distally in the extremities, resection of additional structures such as tendons, nerves, and/or bones is required in a significant portion of cases.[74] Larger tumors are associated with larger resection defects and greater rates of recurrence.[74] Reverse interosseous or radial forearm flaps are options for soft tissue coverage of more proximal defects.[75] However, given the limited regional options, free tissue transfer may be required.

Foot. Much like the hand, sarcomas of the foot are uncommon. Coverage of soft tissue defects of the foot and ankle following sarcoma resection is challenging due to anatomic constraints and the potential impact on functional outcomes. In general, reconstructive considerations are grouped based on whether the defect is on the dorsal or plantar surface of the foot, and thus whether it lies in a weight-bearing or non-weight-bearing area.[76] Reconstruction must take into account the properties of the soft tissues being replaced, the stability of the skeletal structures, and the conservation of sensation in the reconstructed tissue. Skin grafting can be used in small- to medium-sized defects on non-weight-bearing regions but should be avoided in weight-bearing areas. Typically, skin grafting should also be avoided in defects with exposed tendinous structures. However, the use of dermal matrices and NPWT may allow for granulation tissue ingrowth, thus making wounds more amenable to grafting (**Fig. 7**). Reconstruction of weight-bearing regions is particularly difficult. When insensate tissue is used, pressure ulceration is common.[77] On the other hand, sensory reconstruction often results in dysesthesia. In recent years, pedicled and perforator flaps have been used successfully at greater rates for reconstruction of foot and ankle oncologic defects.[78] The sural flap is a good option for the heel and hindfoot and can maintain sensation in the area.[77,79] Plantar surface or distal forefoot defects can be reconstructed with free flaps such as a sensate ALT flap. It is important to advise patients that this will not result in normal sensory function and that the flap will not be as durable as normal plantar skin.

Groin. Unique anatomic considerations in this area include the inguinal ligament and the femoral neurovascular bundle. When resected or divided, the inguinal ligament should be repaired either primarily or with mesh to prevent future hernia formation. Often, local or regional flap coverage is needed for coverage, especially when the neurovascular bundle is exposed or significant dead space exists. If the tumor was in close proximity to vascular structures, radiation may have been used preoperatively or planned in the adjuvant setting. As the inguinal region represents the junction of the torso and thigh, numerous pedicled flap options exist for reconstruction including VRAM and ALT flaps.

Head and Neck. Sarcomas of the head and neck are rare, accounting for only 4% to 10% of all adult sarcomas and only 1% to 2% of all head and neck malignancies.[80,81] In contrast to sarcomas of the torso and extremities, the most common histologic subtypes found in the head and neck are undifferentiated pleomorphic sarcoma, Kaposi sarcoma, fibrosarcoma, and hemangiosarcoma.[1,80,82] Much like other anatomic locations, the mainstay of treatment of tumors of the head and neck is en bloc surgical resection with negative margins; this often poses a problem given the proximity of vital organs and important neurovascular structures as well as the potential for functional and cosmetic morbidity. Incomplete resection with positive margins is an important prognostic factor and leads to poor outcomes in head and neck sarcomas.[83–85] Postoperative radiation may be required in cases with positive margins, and this should be considered at the time of reconstruction. Local and regional tissue transfer options are limited. The trapezius island myocutaneous flap may be an option for

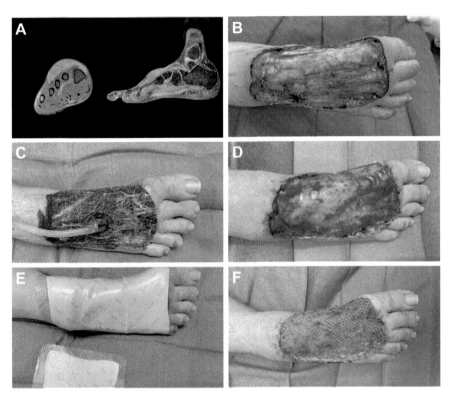

Fig. 7. A 53-year-old woman with an acral myxoinflammatory fibroblastic sarcoma of the dorsum of the foot was referred for surgical evaluation. (*A*) Preoperative MRI showed a 6.8 × 5.4 × 1.2-cm heterogeneous, somewhat ill-defined subcutaneous soft tissue mass of the middorsum of the foot. (*B*) Defect on the dorsum of the foot following wide excision. Tendinous structures are exposed in the wound bed. (*C*) The wound was managed with extensor tenodesis, application of a sheet of bovine collagen bonded to silicone (Integra [Integra LifeSciences, Princeton, NJ, USA]), and an NPWT dressing. (*D*) Ten days after surgery, areas of inosculation can be seen in the matrix after removal of the NPWT dressing. (*E*) After the NPWT dressing is removed, the matrix is protected by a silicone foam dressing until inosculation is complete. (*F*) Once inosculation is complete, the matrix is covered with a split-thickness skin graft.

craniomaxillofacial or neck defects.[86] Free flaps such as ALT, LD, radial forearm, or gracilis flaps are the gold standard for coverage of larger defects.[87–91]

The irradiated field

Given the large number of patients with sarcoma who have or will receive radiation therapy, it is important for the surgeon to know how radiotherapy affects the reconstruction because it may determine what reconstructive option is best. The reconstructing surgeon should play a role in overall treatment planning. Randomized data have demonstrated that preoperative radiation is associated with greater rates of wound complications compared with postoperative radiation.[92] Split-thickness skin grafts are a useful reconstructive adjunct following sarcoma resection, but graft survival on an irradiated bed may be poor.[93] However, survival of the graft may be improved when applied under an NPWT bolster.[94,95] If there is concern regarding healing related to irradiated tissue, free tissue transfer offers the chance to reconstruct the defect with tissue that has not been exposed to radiation. However, even with free tissue transfer, major wound complications still occur in 20% to 45% of cases in these high-risk wounds.[96,97]

SUMMARY

Surgical wide resection remains the mainstay of treatment of sarcomas. However, the advent of effective chemotherapy and radiation therapy has improved outcomes and the rates of limb salvage resection. Given the need for wide resection to achieve negative margins, many wounds are unable to be closed primarily and require plastic surgical reconstruction. Reconstruction should focus on maintaining functional and cosmetic outcomes with minimal postoperative morbidity to the patient. Approaches to reconstruction range from simple techniques such as skin grafting and local rotational flaps all the way to more complex procedures such as free flaps. The reconstructing surgeon is an integral member of the multidisciplinary team and should be actively involved in treatment planning.

CLINICS CARE POINTS

- Multimodality therapy has significantly increased rates of limb salvage resection for sarcoma, often necessitating reconstruction of resection defects.
- Patients are best served by a multidisciplinary approach to resection and reconstruction.
- Following adequate oncologic resection, reconstruction should focus on preserving functional and cosmetic outcomes while minimizing postoperative morbidity.
- The simplest available reconstructive option should be used, but at times a more complex reconstruction may be required.
- Rates of wound complications are increased in irradiated tissues, but this can be minimized with the use of well-vascularized tissue transfer and other adjuncts such as NPWT.

DISCLOSURE

The authors have nothing to disclose.

REFERENCES

1. Brennan MF, Antonescu CR, Moraco N, et al. Lessons learned from the study of 10,000 patients with soft tissue sarcoma. Ann Surg 2014;260(3):416–21 [discussion: 421-2].
2. Siegel RL, Miller KD, Fuchs HE, et al. Cancer statistics, 2021. CA Cancer J Clin 2021;71(1):7–33.
3. Burningham Z, Hashibe M, Spector L, et al. The epidemiology of sarcoma. Clin Sarcoma Res 2012;2(1):14.
4. Abbas JS, Holyoke ED, Moore R, et al. The surgical treatment and outcome of soft-tissue sarcoma. Arch Surg 1981;116(6):765–9.
5. Shiu MH, Castro EB, Hajdu SI, et al. Surgical treatment of 297 soft tissue sarcomas of the lower extremity. Ann Surg 1975;182(5):597–602.
6. Gerner RE, Moore GE, Pickren JW. Soft tissue sarcomas. Ann Surg 1975;181(6):803–8.

7. Italiano A, le Cesne A, Mendiboure J, et al. Prognostic factors and impact of adjuvant treatments on local and metastatic relapse of soft-tissue sarcoma patients in the competing risks setting. Cancer 2014;120(21):3361–9.
8. Sheng JY, Movva S. Systemic therapy for advanced soft tissue sarcoma. Surg Clin North Am 2016;96(5):1141–56.
9. Rosenberg SA, Tepper J, Glatstein E, et al. The treatment of soft-tissue sarcomas of the extremities: prospective randomized evaluations of (1) limb-sparing surgery plus radiation therapy compared with amputation and (2) the role of adjuvant chemotherapy. Ann Surg 1982;196(3):305–15.
10. Yang JC, Chang AE, Baker AR, et al. Randomized prospective study of the benefit of adjuvant radiation therapy in the treatment of soft tissue sarcomas of the extremity. J Clin Oncol 1998;16(1):197–203.
11. Leachman BK, Galloway TJ. The role for radiation therapy in the management of sarcoma. Surg Clin North Am 2016;96(5):1127–39.
12. Lohman RF, Nabawi AS, Reece GP, et al. Soft tissue sarcoma of the upper extremity: a 5-year experience at two institutions emphasizing the role of soft tissue flap reconstruction. Cancer 2002;94(8):2256–64.
13. Karakousis CP, Proimakis C, Walsh DL. Primary soft tissue sarcoma of the extremities in adults. Br J Surg 2005;82(9). https://doi.org/10.1002/bjs.1800820919.
14. Chao AH, Mayerson JL, Chandawarkar R, et al. Surgical management of soft tissue sarcomas: extremity sarcomas. J Surg Oncol 2015;111(5):540–5.
15. Malek F, Somerson JS, Mitchel S, et al. Does limb-salvage surgery offer patients better quality of life and functional capacity than amputation? Clin Orthop Relat Res 2012;470(7):2000–6.
16. Nagarajan R, Neglia JP, Clohisy DR, et al. Limb salvage and amputation in survivors of pediatric lower-extremity bone tumors: what are the long-term implications? J Clin Oncol 2002;20(22):4493–501.
17. Nelson JA, Fischer JP, Grover R, et al. Vein grafting your way out of trouble: Examining the utility and efficacy of vein grafts in microsurgery. J Plast Reconstr Aesthet Surg 2015;68(6):830–6.
18. Pederson WC, Grome L. Microsurgical reconstruction of the lower extremity. Semin Plast Surg 2019;33(1):54–8.
19. Dibbs R, Grome L, Pederson WC. Free tissue transfer for upper extremity reconstruction. Semin Plast Surg 2019;33(1):17–23.
20. Moreira-Gonzalez A, Djohan R, Lohman R. Considerations surrounding reconstruction after resection of musculoskeletal sarcomas. Cleveland Clinic J Med 2010;77(Suppl 1):S18–22.
21. Morii T, Mochizuki K, Takushima A, et al. Soft tissue reconstruction using vascularized tissue transplantation following resection of musculoskeletal sarcoma: evaluation of oncologic and functional outcomes in 55 cases. Ann Plast Surg 2009;62(3):252–7.
22. Wang D, Bosch W, Roberge D, et al. RTOG sarcoma radiation oncologists reach consensus on gross tumor volume and clinical target volume on computed tomographic images for preoperative radiotherapy of primary soft tissue sarcoma of extremity in Radiation Therapy Oncology Group studies. Int J Radiat Oncol Biol Phys 2011;81(4):e525–8.
23. Cannon CP, Ballo MT, Zagars GK, et al. Complications of combined modality treatment of primary lower extremity soft-tissue sarcomas. Cancer 2006; 107(10):2455–61.
24. Miller ED, Xu-Welliver M, Haglund KE. The role of modern radiation therapy in the management of extremity sarcomas. J Surg Oncol 2015;111(5):599–603.

25. Punzalan M, Hyden G. The role of physical therapy and occupational therapy in the rehabilitation of pediatric and adolescent patients with osteosarcoma. Cancer Treat Res 2009. https://doi.org/10.1007/978-1-4419-0284-9_20.
26. Tobias K, Gillis T. Rehabilitation of the sarcoma patient-enhancing the recovery and functioning of patients undergoing management for extremity soft tissue sarcomas. J Surg Oncol 2015;111(5):615–21.
27. Smith SR. Rehabilitation strategies and outcomes of the sarcoma patient. Phys Med Rehabil Clin N Am 2017;28(1):171–80.
28. Janis JE, Kwon RK, Attinger CE. The new reconstructive ladder: modifications to the traditional model. Plast Reconstr Surg 2011;127(Suppl 1):205S–12S.
29. Bennett N, Choudhary S. Why climb a ladder when you can take the elevator? Plast Reconstr Surg 2000;105(6):2266.
30. Endara M, Masden D, Goldstein J, et al. The role of chronic and perioperative glucose management in high-risk surgical closures: a case for tighter glycemic control. Plast Reconstr Surg 2013;132(4):996–1004.
31. Arnold PG, Pairolero PC. Chest-wall reconstruction: an account of 500 consecutive patients. Plast Reconstr Surg 1996;98(5):804–10.
32. Momeni A, Kovach SJ. Important considerations in chest wall reconstruction. J Surg Oncol 2016;113(8):913–22.
33. Mahabir RC, Butler CE. Stabilization of the chest wall: autologous and alloplastic reconstructions. Semin Plast Surg 2011;25(1):34–42.
34. Shah NR, Ayyala HS, Tran BNN, et al. Outcomes in chest wall reconstruction using methyl methacrylate prostheses: a review of the literature and case series utilizing a novel approach with biologic mesh. J Reconstr Microsurg 2019;35(8):575–86.
35. Hameed A, Akhtar S, Naqvi A, et al. Reconstruction of complex chest wall defects by using polypropylene mesh and a pedicled latissimus dorsi flap: a 6-year experience. J Plast Reconstr Aesthet Surg 2008;61(6):628–35.
36. Losken A, Thourani VH, Carlson GW, et al. A reconstructive algorithm for plastic surgery following extensive chest wall resection. Br J Plast Surg 2004;57(4):295–302.
37. Weyant MJ, Bains MS, Venkatraman E, et al. Results of chest wall resection and reconstruction with and without rigid prosthesis. Ann Thorac Surg 2006;81(1):279–85.
38. Hultman CS, Culbertson JH, Jones GE, et al. Thoracic reconstruction with the omentum: indications, complications, and results. Ann Plast Surg 2001;46(3):242–9.
39. Williams KJ, Hayes AJ. A guide to oncological management of soft tissue tumours of the abdominal wall. Hernia 2014;18(1):91–7.
40. Stojadinovic A, Hoos A, Karpoff HM, et al. Soft tissue tumors of the abdominal wall: analysis of disease patterns and treatment. Arch Surg 2001;136(1):70–9.
41. Breuing K, Butler CE, Ferzoco S, et al, Ventral Hernia Working Group. Incisional ventral hernias: review of the literature and recommendations regarding the grading and technique of repair. Surgery 2010;148(3):544–58.
42. Khansa I, Janis JE. Modern reconstructive techniques for abdominal wall defects after oncologic resection. J Surg Oncol 2015;111(5):587–98.
43. Mericli AF, Baumann DP, Butler CE. Reconstruction of the abdominal wall after oncologic resection: defect classification and management strategies. Plast Reconstr Surg 2018;142(3 Suppl):187S–96S.
44. Luijendijk RW, Hop WC, van den Tol MP, et al. A comparison of suture repair with mesh repair for incisional hernia. N Engl J Med 2000;343(6):392–8.

45. Booth JH, Garvey PB, Baumann DP, et al. Primary fascial closure with mesh reinforcement is superior to bridged mesh repair for abdominal wall reconstruction. J Am Coll Surg 2013;217(6):999–1009.
46. D'Arpa S, Toia F, Pirrello R, et al. Propeller flaps: a review of indications, technique, and results. Biomed Res Int 2014;2014:986829.
47. Scaglioni MF, Giuseppe AD, Chang EI. Propeller flap reconstruction of abdominal defects: review of the literature and case report. Microsurgery 2015;35(1):72–8.
48. Kuo YR, Kuo MH, Lutz BS, et al. One-stage reconstruction of large midline abdominal wall defects using a composite free anterolateral thigh flap with vascularized fascia lata. Ann Surg 2004;239(3):352–8.
49. Oh J, Oh JS, Eun SC. Extensive full thickness abdominal wall reconstruction using anterolateral thigh compound flap modifications. Microsurgery 2020;40(3): 337–42.
50. chan WF, Jain V, Celik N, et al. Have we found an ideal soft-tissue flap? An experience with 672 anterolateral thigh flaps. Plast Reconstr Surg 2002;109(7): 2219–26 [discussion: 2227-30].
51. Suresh V, Gao J, Jung SH, et al. The role of reconstructive surgery after skeletal and soft tissue sarcoma resection. Ann Plast Surg 2018;80(6S Suppl 6):S372–6.
52. Zaretski A, Amir A, Meller I, et al. Free fibula long bone reconstruction in orthopedic oncology: a surgical algorithm for reconstructive options. Plast Reconstr Surg 2004;113(7):1989–2000.
53. Chen CM, Disa JJ, Lee HY, et al. Reconstruction of extremity long bone defects after sarcoma resection with vascularized fibula flaps: a 10-year review. Plast Reconstr Surg 2007;119(3):915–24 [discussion: 925-6].
54. Behnam AB, Chen CM, Pusic AL, et al. The pedicled latissimus dorsi flap for shoulder reconstruction after sarcoma resection. Ann Surg Oncol 2007;14(5): 1591–5.
55. Kim JS, Lee JS, Yoon JO, et al. Reconstruction of the shoulder region using a pedicled latissimus dorsi flap after resection of soft tissue due to sarcoma. J Plast Reconstr Aesthet Surg 2009;62(9):1215–8.
56. Jones NF, Jarrahy R, Kaufman MR. Pedicled and free radial forearm flaps for reconstruction of the elbow, wrist, and hand. Plast Reconstr Surg 2008;121(3): 887–98.
57. Kim JY, Youssef A, Subramanian V, et al. Upper extremity reconstruction following resection of soft tissue sarcomas: a functional outcomes analysis. Ann Surg Oncol 2004;11(10):921–7.
58. Oh E, Seo SW, Han KJ. A longitudinal study of functional outcomes in patients with limb salvage surgery for soft tissue sarcoma. Sarcoma 2018;2018:6846275.
59. Labow BI, Rosen H, Greene AK, et al. Soft tissue sarcomas of the hand: functional reconstruction and outcome analysis. Hand (NY) 2008;3(3):229–36.
60. MacArthur IR, McInnes CW, Dalke KR, et al. Patient reported outcomes following lower extremity soft tissue sarcoma resection with microsurgical preservation of ambulation. J Reconstr Microsurg 2019;35(3):168–75.
61. Petukhova TA, Navrazhina K, Minkis K. V-Y Hemi-keystone advancement flap: a novel and simplified reconstructive modification. Plast Reconstr Surg Glob open 2020;8(2):e2654.
62. Rao AL, Janna RK. Keystone flap: versatile flap for reconstruction of limb defects. J Clin Diagn Res 2015;9(3):PC05-7.
63. Riccio CA, Chang J, Henderson JT, et al. Keystone flaps: physiology, types, and clinical applications. Ann Plast Surg 2019;83(2):226–31.

64. Daigeler A, Simidjiiska-Belyaeva M, Drücke D, et al. The versatility of the pedicled vertical rectus abdominis myocutaneous flap in oncologic patients. Langenbeck's Arch Surg 2011;396(8):1271-9.

65. Parrett BM, Winograd JM, Garfein ES, et al. The vertical and extended rectus abdominis myocutaneous flap for irradiated thigh and groin defects. Plast Reconstr Surg 2008;122(1):171-7.

66. Khalil HH, El-Ghoneimy A, Farid Y, et al. Modified vertical rectus abdominis musculocutaneous flap for limb salvage procedures in proximal lower limb musculoskeletal sarcomas. Sarcoma 2008;2008:781408.

67. Friji MT, Suri MP, Shankhdhar VK, et al. Pedicled anterolateral thigh flap: a versatile flap for difficult regional soft tissue reconstruction. Ann Plast Surg 2010;64(4):458-61.

68. Ellabban MA, Awad AI, Hallock GG. Perforator-pedicled propeller flaps for lower extremity reconstruction. Semin Plast Surg 2020;34(3):200-6.

69. Walton Z, Armstrong M, Traven S, et al. Pedicled rotational medial and lateral gastrocnemius flaps: surgical technique. J Am Acad Orthop Surg 2017;25(11):744-51.

70. Almeida MF, da Costa PR, Okawa RY. Reverse-flow island sural flap. Plast Reconstr Surg 2002;109(2):583-91.

71. Kozusko SD, Liu X, Riccio CA, et al. Selecting a free flap for soft tissue coverage in lower extremity reconstruction. Injury 2019;50(Suppl 5):S32-9.

72. Medina MA, Salinas HM, Eberlin KR, et al. Modified free radial forearm fascia flap reconstruction of lower extremity and foot wounds: optimal contour and minimal donor-site morbidity. J Reconstr Microsurg 2014;30(8):515-22.

73. Lee MJ, Yun IS, Rah DK, et al. Lower extremity reconstruction using vastus lateralis myocutaneous flap versus anterolateral thigh fasciocutaneous flap. Arch Plast Surg 2012;39(4):367-75.

74. Dadras M, Steinau HU, Goertz O, et al. Limb preserving surgery for soft-tissue sarcoma in the hand: a retrospective study of 51 cases. J Hand Surg Eur Vol 2020;45(6):629-35.

75. Mirous MP, Coulet B, Chammas M, et al. Extensive limb-sparing surgery with reconstruction for sarcoma of the hand and wrist. Orthopaedics Traumatol Surg Res 2016;102(4):467-72.

76. Ring A, Kirchhoff P, Goertz O, et al. Reconstruction of soft-tissue defects at the foot and ankle after oncological resection. Front Surg 2016;3:15.

77. Tan O, Aydin OE, Demir R, et al. Neurotized sural flap: an alternative in sensory reconstruction of the foot and ankle defects. Microsurgery 2015;35(3):183-9.

78. Mallett KE, Houdek MT, Honig RL, et al. Comparison of flap reconstruction for soft tissue sarcomas of the foot and ankle. J Surg Oncol 2021;124(7):995-1001.

79. Zhu YL, Wang Y, He XQ, et al. Foot and ankle reconstruction: an experience on the use of 14 different flaps in 226 cases. Microsurgery 2013;33(8):600-4.

80. Peng KA, Grogan T, Wang MB. Head and neck sarcomas: analysis of the SEER database. Otolaryngol Head Neck Surg 2014;151(4):627-33.

81. Kraus DH. Sarcomas of the head and neck. Curr Oncol Rep 2002;4(1):68-75.

82. Bentz BG, Singh B, Woodruff J, et al. Head and neck soft tissue sarcomas: a multivariate analysis of outcomes. Ann Surg Oncol 2004;11(6):619-28.

83. Patel SG, Shaha AR, Shah JP. Soft tissue sarcomas of the head and neck: an update. Am J Otolaryngol 2001;22(1):2-18.

84. Kraus DH, Dubner S, Harrison LB, et al. Prognostic factors for recurrence and survival in head and neck soft tissue sarcomas. Cancer 1994;74(2):697-702.

85. le Vay J, O'Sullivan B, Catton C, et al. An assessment of prognostic factors in soft-tissue sarcoma of the head and neck. Arch Otolaryngol Head Neck Surg 1994; 120(9):981–6.
86. Chen WL, Liu YM, Zhou B, et al. En bloc resection and reconstruction in patients with advanced recurrent nasopharyngeal carcinoma and radiation-induced sarcoma of the head and neck. Int J Oral Maxillofac Surg 2021;50(6):711–7.
87. Ehrl D, Brueggemann A, Broer PN, et al. Scalp reconstruction after malignant tumor resection: an analysis and algorithm. J Neurol Surg B Skull Base 2020; 81(02):149–57.
88. Simunovic F, Eisenhardt SU, Penna V, et al. Microsurgical reconstruction of oncological scalp defects in the elderly. J Plast Reconstr Aesthet Surg 2016;69(7): 912–9.
89. Lutz BS. Aesthetic and functional advantages of the anterolateral thigh flap in reconstruction of tumor-related scalp defects. Microsurgery 2002;22(6):258–64.
90. Lipa JE, Butler CE. Enhancing the outcome of free latissimus dorsi muscle flap reconstruction of scalp defects. Head Neck 2004;26(1):46–53.
91. Sweeny L, Eby B, Magnuson JS, et al. Reconstruction of scalp defects with the radial forearm free flap. Head Neck Oncol 2012;4:21.
92. O'Sullivan B, Davis AM, Turcotte R, et al. Preoperative versus postoperative radiotherapy in soft-tissue sarcoma of the limbs: a randomised trial. Lancet (London, England) 2002;359(9325):2235–41.
93. Bui DT, Chunilal A, Mehrara BJ, et al. Outcome of split-thickness skin grafts after external beam radiotherapy. Ann Plast Surg 2004;52(6):551–6 [discussion: 557].
94. Senchenkov A, Petty PM, Knoetgen J, et al. Outcomes of skin graft reconstructions with the use of Vacuum Assisted Closure (VAC(R)) dressing for irradiated extremity sarcoma defects. World J Surg Oncol 2007;5:138.
95. Bedi M, King DM, DeVries J, et al. Does vacuum-assisted closure reduce the risk of wound complications in patients with lower extremity sarcomas treated with preoperative radiation? Clin Orthopaedics Relat Res 2019;477(4):768–74.
96. Barwick WJ, Goldberg JA, Scully SP, et al. Vascularized tissue transfer for closure of irradiated wounds after soft tissue sarcoma resection. Ann Surg 1992;216(5): 591–5.
97. Tseng JF, Ballo MT, Langstein HN, et al. The effect of preoperative radiotherapy and reconstructive surgery on wound complications after resection of extremity soft-tissue sarcomas. Ann Surg Oncol 2006;13(9):1209–15.

Retroperitoneal Sarcomas
Histology Is Everything

Michael K. Turgeon, MD[a], Kenneth Cardona, MD[b],*

KEYWORDS

- Retroperitoneal sarcoma • Histiotype • Surgery • Multimodality therapy
- Active surveillance

KEY POINTS

- Retroperitoneal sarcomas represent approximately 15% of all soft tissue sarcomas cases seen in the Unites States.
- Surgical wide resection remains the only curative treatment option; however, the frequent proximity of the tumor to critical organs and vascular structures complicates the ability to obtain widely negative surgical margins.
- Tumor biology, disease presentation, treatment options, patterns of recurrence, and surveillance protocols vary depending on the sarcoma histologic subtype.
- Histologic subtype-specific multimodality therapy is emerging as the preferred treatment strategy, guided by the expertise of a multidisciplinary tumor board at specialized sarcoma referral centers.

INTRODUCTION

Although soft tissue sarcomas account for less than 1% of all adult cancers in the United States, retroperitoneal sarcomas (RPS) encompass only 16% of these cases.[1] With more than 100 histologic soft tissue sarcoma subtypes identified to date, any of which can occur in the retroperitoneum, it is important to note that most RPS cases predominantly involve 3 histologies: liposarcoma, leiomyosarcoma, and solitary fibrous tumor (SFT).[2] However, each of these histologies has considerable variability in disease presentation, progression, and oncologic outcomes. As a result, the prevailing treatment paradigm has evolved from a uniform approach to one more tailored to histologic subtype.[3]

Liposarcomas are adipocytic tumors that arise within the retroperitoneal fat and represent the most common RPS histologic subtype (nearly 50%). They are further

[a] Division of Surgical Oncology, Department of Surgery, Winship Cancer Institute, Emory University, 1365 Clifton Road, NE, Building B, Suite 4100, Office 4201, Atlanta, GA 30322, USA;
[b] Division of Surgical Oncology, Department of Surgery, Winship Cancer Institute, Emory University, 550 Peachtree Street, NE, 9th Floor, Suite 900, Atlanta, GA 30308, USA
* Corresponding author.
E-mail address: ken.cardona@emory.edu

Surg Clin N Am 102 (2022) 601–614
https://doi.org/10.1016/j.suc.2022.04.004
0039-6109/22/© 2022 Elsevier Inc. All rights reserved.
surgical.theclinics.com

categorized as well-differentiated, dedifferentiated, or mixed well-differentiated/ dedifferentiated tumors (**Figs. 1–3**). Liposarcomas typically localize to either the right or left retroperitoneal space and can occupy the hemiabdomen displacing the kidney, colon, and/or pancreas medially. They can also grow to the point where the tumor crosses midline and occupies the contralateral hemiabdomen. It is important to note the diagnosis of undifferentiated pleomorphic sarcoma/malignant fibrous histiocytoma in the retroperitoneum most likely represents a dedifferentiated liposarcoma that can now be effectively diagnosed with molecular assessment for MDM2 amplification. An exception to this can be a tumor that is confined within the retroperitoneal musculature (eg, psoas muscle). The other liposarcoma subtypes, such as myxoid/ round cell and pleomorphic, rarely occur primarily in the retroperitoneum.[4] From a tumor biology standpoint, well-differentiated (low-grade) liposarcomas have a predisposition for local recurrence with 5-year local recurrence rates of 18% to 41% but do not metastasize to distant sites (eg, lung or liver; **Table 1**). In contrast, dedifferentiated (high-grade) liposarcomas often develop both local and distant metastases with 5-year local and distant recurrence rates of 45% to 58% and 25% to 44%, respectively.[5,6]

Retroperitoneal I left leiomyosarcomas arise from smooth muscle, most commonly from the major venous vasculature of the retroperitoneum (vena cava or iliac/renal/ gonadal veins) and represent the second most common (10%–15%) histologic subtype encountered in the retroperitoneum (**Fig. 4**). Specifically, these tumors originate from the wall of the vein and can demonstrate both exophytic growth from the vessel wall maintaining the patency of the blood vessel or completely obliterate the vessel lumen. When discussing retroperitoneal leiomyosarcomas, it is important to note that uterine leiomyosarcomas are considered gynecologic sarcomas and are not managed in the same way as a true retroperitoneal leiomyosarcoma. Retroperitoneal leiomyosarcomas are typically high-grade, aggressive tumors that have low rates of local recurrence (10%) but high rates of distant metastatic disease, exceeding 50% at 5 years.[5,6]

SFTs are mesenchymal tumors that can arise anywhere in the body and account for approximately 5% of RPS (**Fig. 5**).[5] They have a more favorable prognosis given low rates for both local recurrence (7%–9% at 5 years) as well as distant metastases (18%–35% at 5 years).[5–7]

Given the broad spectrum of diseases that can mimic RPS, it is critical for clinicians to recognize tumors presenting in the retroperitoneum that resemble, yet are not an RPS. These include lymphoma, primary germ cell tumors, metastatic testicular

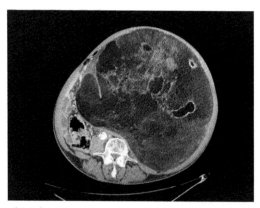

Fig. 1. Axial image of a left-sided retroperitoneal well-differentiated liposarcoma.

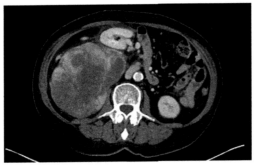

Fig. 2. Axial image of a right-sided retroperitoneal dedifferentiated liposarcoma.

cancer, adrenal tumors, and renal tumors. Because there can be considerable overlap between the radiographic appearance of these tumors and RPS, a tissue diagnosis is critical. The challenge of histopathologic assessment and diagnosis emphasizes the importance of enlisting expert pathologic assessment at specialized centers.

The complexity of RPS management has resulted in considerable debate regarding the optimal therapeutic approach. Although surgical resection remains the cornerstone of treatment, the decision to pursue multimodality therapy, including chemotherapy and/or radiation therapy, relies on patient-specific and tumor-specific factors that require multidisciplinary discussion. The following is a broad overview of current management guidelines and highlights emerging treatment strategies.

CLINICAL PRESENTATION

The most common presenting symptom for RPS patients is a painless, enlarging mass. Patients are generally asymptomatic until the mass effect from the tumor's growth is significant enough to compress or impinge on surrounding organs, which may result in ambiguous complaints such as abdominal discomfort or fullness, early satiety, and/or weight loss. This is typically, but not exclusively, seen with liposarcomas. In rare cases, patients can present with lower extremity swelling if venous outflow is impeded, which is not uncommon with caval or iliac vein leiomyosarcomas. Given the significant potential space of the retroperitoneum, an RPS can often exceed 15 cm in size at initial evaluation with 70% of tumors larger than 10 cm.[8]

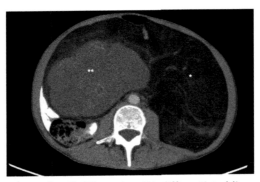

Fig. 3. Axial image of mixed well-differentiated/dedifferentiated liposarcoma with a left-sided well-differentiated component (*asterisk*) and a right-sided dedifferentiated component (*double asterisk*).

	Table 1 Recurrence patterns and survival based on histologic subtype			
Histologic Subtype	Percent Makeup of RPS	5-y Local Recurrence Rate	5-y Distant Recurrence Rate	5-y OS
Liposarcoma (well-differentiated)	28%–34%	18%–41%	<1%	66%–92%
Liposarcoma (dedifferentiated)	23%–32%	45%–58%	25%–44%	42%–53%
Leiomyosarcoma	15%–23%	6%–18%	51%–56%	56%–58%
SFT	5%–7%	7%–9%	18%–35%	78%–84%

Percent makeup, local recurrence, distant recurrence, and 5-y OS rates by histologic subtype.[50]

DIAGNOSIS
Imaging

Contrast-enhanced computed tomography (CT) is the gold standard for the diagnostic evaluation of RPS, allowing for assessment of the local extent of the tumor and potential sites of metastatic disease. This is in contrast to the work-up of truncal/extremity sarcomas, where magnetic resonance imaging is the preferred modality. On cross-sectional imaging of the abdomen and pelvis, the location/epicenter of the tumor, the extent of tumor burden, interface of the tumor with surrounding abdominal viscera, and associated vasculature should be noted to inform management decisions, including operative planning and the potential role for multimodality therapy. Moreover, the addition of a staging chest CT is recommended, particularly for high-grade RPS, where up to 14% of patients present with synchronous pulmonary metastases.[9]

Core Needle Biopsy

Once an RPS is suspected, the National Comprehensive Cancer Network (NCCN) guidelines recommend referral to a high-volume, specialized sarcoma center.[10] A preoperative CT-guided core needle biopsy with a coaxial needle and subsequent evaluation by an experienced sarcoma pathologist is critical. Almond and colleagues[11] reported an overall concordance of core needle biopsy with final pathology following resection of 67.2%, with dedifferentiated liposarcomas accounting for most of the discrepancies. Given the challenges associated with histologic assessment, a definitive diagnosis often requires a combination of immunohistochemistry, molecular testing,

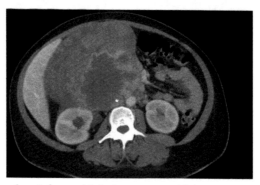

Fig. 4. Axial image of an infrarenal inferior vena caval leiomyosarcoma (*asterisk*: inferior vena cava).

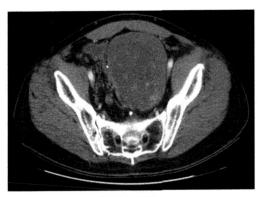

Fig. 5. Axial image of a retroperitoneal/pelvic SFT.

and cytogenetic techniques to corroborate clinical and radiological findings—emphasizing the importance of multidisciplinary tumor board discussion of these cases with dedicated radiologists and pathologists. Moreover, core needle biopsy is safe and is associated with few complications, especially with modern sampling techniques. A recent retrospective review of 358 patients by Berger-Richardson and colleagues[12] reported very low rates of core needle biopsy complications: 2% minor bleeding with no transfusion, 0.8% significant pain, 0.3% unplanned hospital admission, and 0.3% pneumothorax. Although there is some concern for needle-tract seeding, the risk is minimal because recent retrospective studies report rates of less than 1%.[13,14] When technically possible, the trajectory of the core needle biopsy should avoid the free intra-abdominal space. Finally, histologic subtype offers the opportunity to guide preoperative treatment approaches. Specifically, for those with resectable disease, patients may be candidates for neoadjuvant therapy. Overall, the benefits of a preoperative tissue diagnosis outweigh any potential harm.

Staging

The eighth edition of the American Joint Committee on Cancer (AJCC)/Union for International Cancer Control, among the most widely used classification systems, provides staging recommendations.[15] However, the fact that histologic subtype, an established predictor of prognosis, is not accounted for limits its applicability.

More recently, nomograms have been used to better predict the survival and risk of recurrence. Nomograms typically include patient-specific clinicopathologic factors, thereby offering a more accurate prognostic model to better inform patients and clinicians. In patients with primary RPS, Gronchi and colleagues[16] developed a nomogram (SARCULATOR) for predicting 3-year and 5-year overall survival (OS) and disease-free survival (DFS) with covariates that included age, tumor size, grade, histologic subtype, multifocality, quality of surgery, and radiation therapy. This nomogram for RPS has been endorsed by the AJCC.

TREATMENT APPROACHES

Historically, the diversity of RPS histology-specific biologic behavior has limited our ability to adopt a standardized treatment approach. However, in the past 20 years, an enhanced understanding of RPS biology and the importance of patient selection, surgical technique, and perioperative management has modified potentially curative treatment approaches and improved long-term oncologic outcomes. Progress has been possible through the concerted efforts of multi-institutional cooperative groups, specifically the Transatlantic Australasian Retroperitoneal Sarcoma Working Group (TARPSWG). TARPSWG is an international consortium formed in 2013 to help shape the guiding principles of the management of RPS patients, emphasizing the importance of collaboration in the treatment of rare cancers.[17]

Currently, multimodality therapy remains a subject of considerable debate. Although well studied in truncal/extremity sarcomas, there is limited data supporting its applicability in the treatment of RPS patients. As a result, the role for radiation therapy and/or chemotherapy should be discussed in the context of a multidisciplinary team at a specialized sarcoma center.

Specialized Sarcoma Centers

Given the significant heterogeneity of RPS histologic subtypes and the complexity of their surgical management, current guidelines recommend patients with RPS be referred to a specialized sarcoma center, particularly for initial evaluation, as the best chance of cure is at the index operation.[17,18] Doing so streamlines care delivery, permits early involvement of a multidisciplinary team, and access to potential multimodality therapies, including clinical trial enrollment.[19] Large retrospective studies by Blay and colleagues[20] and Keung and colleagues[21] have demonstrated improved oncologic outcomes for patients treated at high-volume versus low-volume centers. Contributing factors include increased surgeon volume, experience of the treatment team, and oncology support services.

Surgery

For localized, primary RPS, surgical resection remains the cornerstone of treatment and the only chance of cure. Accordingly, the completeness of resection is a major predictor of both recurrence and survival.[22,23] In a multi-institutional study that included 1942 patients who underwent curative-intent resection between 2002 and 2017, Callegaro and colleagues[24] noted that the combined R0 (macroscopic or microscopic cancer not demonstrable at the resection margin) and R1 (microscopic margins positive for tumor) resection rate exceeded 93% for the entire study and 5-year OS for each of the treatment periods increased over time (61.2 [95% CI 56.4%–66.3%], 67.0% [95% CI 63.2%–71.0%], and 71.9% [95% CI 67.7%–76.1%], respectively). A 2017 National Cancer Database (NCDB) study of 4015 patients with RPS by Stahl and colleagues[25] noted improved OS in patients who achieved R0 resections as compared with R1 and R2 (macroscopic margins positive for tumor) resections. In the modern era of sarcoma management, these series highlight the importance of determining resectability and the impact of oncologically appropriate tumor resection at the time of the index operation on recurrence and survival.

The *optimal* surgical approach for RPS would allow for a wide margin of resection. However, this is often challenging given the abutment or frank invasion of tumor into adjacent organs. Most experts agree that significant involvement of the aorta (specifically at the level of the celiac axis and superior mesenteric artery), liver hilum, and/or spinal cord precludes surgery.[26] Moreover, patients with evidence of distant metastases or multifocal intra-abdominal disease will likely not benefit from surgery.[27]

On entering the abdomen via a midline laparotomy incision, the surgeon should assess for sarcomatosis. If there is no evidence of peritoneal implants, then the retroperitoneum should be inspected before tumor mobilization. In cases where there is tumor involvement of adjacent organs and/or structures (eg, kidney, colon, pancreas, spleen, psoas muscle, and/or diaphragm), an en bloc surgical resection with the extent of multivisceral resection being tailored to the specific histology should be performed with the intent being to achieve a grossly negative margin of resection (**Fig. 6A**). This approach can improve local disease control and has been associated with improved long-term oncologic outcomes.[28,29] Additionally, vascular involvement is *not* an absolute contraindication to surgery, and select patients may benefit from major vascular resection/reconstruction of the infrarenal aorta, vena cava, and/or iliac vessels (**Fig. 7**).[30] As stated above, retroperitoneal leiomyosarcomas primarily originate from the major venous blood vessels (inferior vena cava, renal veins, iliac veins, gonadal veins, and so forth) Consequently, depending on the vein of origin and whether or not the vessel is still patent, simple ligation versus reconstruction (patch repair or interposition graft) may be required.

More recently, *extended* or *compartmental resection*, which entails resecting all associated organs/structures on the ipsilateral side of the tumor, irrespective of tumor involvement, has been used at some specialized sarcoma centers (see **Fig. 6B**).[31] This approach is specifically considered for a retroperitoneal liposarcoma given that clearance of all retroperitoneal fat from the diaphragm to the iliac vessels can remove

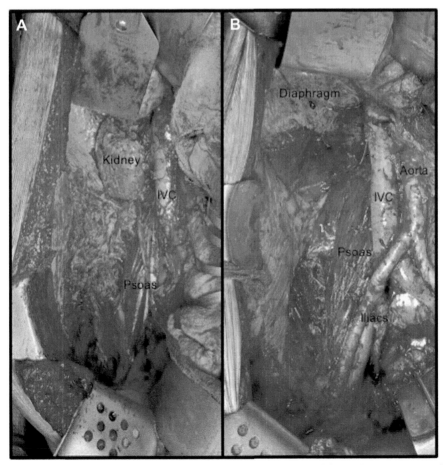

Fig. 6. (*A*) En bloc resection with clearance of right retroperitoneal fat with preservation of the right kidney; (*B*): Compartmental resection with clearance of right retroperitoneal fat (IVC: inferior vena cava).[Note: Change panels as changed in Fig. 6]

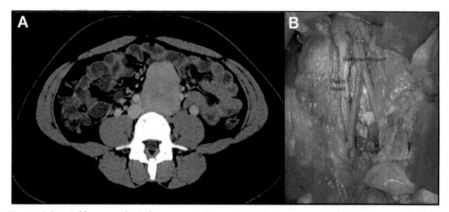

Fig. 7. (A) Axial image of a left common iliac vein leiomyosarcoma with involvement of the aortic bifurcation. (B) Major vascular resection with patch repair of the vena cava and placement of an aorto-bi-iliac interposition graft.

clinically inapparent multifocal disease as well as minimize confusion regarding possible local recurrence on postoperative surveillance imaging. In a series of 331 patients with low-to-intermediate-grade RPS, Gronchi and colleagues[32] demonstrated improved local control and 5-year OS in patients who underwent extended resection. However, this approach remains a subject of continued discussion among sarcoma surgeons. An en bloc resection, where all ipsilateral retroperitoneal fat is still cleared, but with organ preservation in the absence of frank invasion in order to achieve an R0/R1 margin without extended resection is still frequently pursued at most sarcoma centers (**Fig. 8**).

Neoadjuvant Therapy

Given that different histologic subtypes have varying propensities for local recurrence (eg, well-differentiated liposarcomas) or distant metastatic disease (eg, dedifferentiated liposarcomas and leiomyosarcomas), prospectively examining the impact of multimodality therapy, particularly in the neoadjuvant setting, presents a significant opportunity for the treatment of high-risk patients.

Radiation Therapy

Historically, extrapolating from literature for extremity soft tissue sarcomas, radiation therapy in combination with surgery for RPS has been variably used given its potential to reduce local recurrences, which can cause mortality in some RPS patients.[33–35] Retrospective series have supported the use of neoadjuvant radiation therapy for patients with localized, resectable RPS. In a propensity score-matched NCDB study that included patients with localized, primary RPS, Nussbaum and colleagues[36] reported that neoadjuvant radiation therapy was associated with improved OS as compared with surgery alone (HR 0.70, 95% CI 0.59–0.82, $P < .01$). Hence, many sarcoma centers have incorporated neoadjuvant radiation therapy in their multidisciplinary management of RPS.

Recently, the international phase 3 randomized controlled STRASS trial (EORTC 62092) compared preoperative radiation therapy plus surgery to surgery alone for 266 patients with localized, primary RPS at 31 centers.[37] This was deemed a negative trial because there was no statistically significant improvement in abdominal

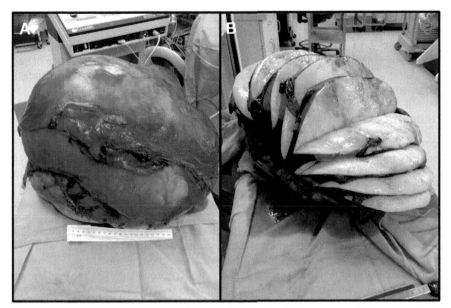

Fig. 8. (A) Gross resection specimen of a well-differentiated liposarcoma; (B) Sectioned well-differentiated liposarcoma.

recurrence-free survival (ARFS); 3-year ARFS was 60.4% in the preoperative radiation therapy group versus 58.7% in the surgery group (P = .95). This study also showed that radiation therapy has a limited role in the treatment of high-grade sarcoma histologies (G3 dedifferentiated liposarcoma and leiomyosarcoma). I post interestingly, in a post hoc subset analysis of patients with well-differentiated liposarcoma and low-grade (G1) dedifferentiated liposarcoma, there was an improvement in ARFS, suggesting there might be a role for preoperative radiation therapy for specific RPS histology. Nevertheless, this subset analysis was neither planned nor appropriately powered; therefore, one must take caution in drawing any definitive conclusions. These data further highlight the importance of multidisciplinary discussion of these complex cases.

In the adjuvant (postoperative) setting, there is no conclusive data to support the routine use of radiation therapy after curative-intent resection.[38,39] This is reflected in the TARPSWG consensus guidelines that recommends against adjuvant radiation therapy in RPS patients.[17]

Chemotherapy

The role for neoadjuvant chemotherapy for RPS remains unclear, although there might be some utility in chemosensitive histologies with a high risk of distant metastases: dedifferentiated liposarcoma, leiomyosarcoma, synovial sarcoma, and malignant SFT. Existing evidence for considering neoadjuvant chemotherapy is largely derived from randomized controlled trials for truncal/extremity soft tissue sarcomas or retrospective studies, the latter of which have conflicting results due to a lack of histology-specific inclusion criteria.[40–43] Similar to other malignancies, neoadjuvant chemotherapy provides an in vivo assessment of the tumor treatment response, addresses micrometastatic disease early, and potentially increases rates of curative resection. To evaluate the role of neoadjuvant chemotherapy for RPS patients with the highest risk for metastatic disease, namely high-grade dedifferentiated liposarcoma and high-grade leiomyosarcoma, the EORTC 1809 STRASS II randomized control trial will compare neoadjuvant chemotherapy plus surgery to surgery alone with the primary outcome of DFS (NCT04031677). Hence, the current consideration of neoadjuvant chemotherapy should be carefully discussed in the context of a multidisciplinary tumor board on a case-by-case basis.

RECURRENCE

Locoregional, distant, and combined recurrences can lead to significant morbidity and mortality for RPS patients; this is largely dictated by the tumor biology and histologic subtype (**Fig. 9**).[2,5,44] In a multi-institutional study of 498 patients with RPS, Chouliaras and colleagues[45] reported overall recurrence rates of 25.3% for locoregional, 16.5% for distant, and 14.5% combined locoregional/distant. Comparing patients who recurred to those who did not, the 5-year OS rate was 51.8% versus 83.9%, respectively ($P < .01$). Furthermore, the ability to achieve an R0 resection margin decreased with each successive operation for a locoregional recurrence: 57%, 33%, and 14% following the first, second, and third recurrence resection, respectively.[46] Given the importance of the index surgery for achieving an R0 resection margin, the involvement of an experienced sarcoma treatment team to optimize the initial surgery is crucial.[47,48] For locoregionally recurrent disease, the role of surgery is beyond the scope of this review article and is an area of ongoing investigation that merits evaluation at a dedicated sarcoma center.

SURVEILLANCE

For RPS patients who underwent a curative-intent resection, current NCCN guidelines recommend a physical examination and contrast-enhanced cross-sectional imaging of the abdomen and pelvis every 3 to 6 months for the first 2 to 3 years, then every 6 months for the next 2 years, then yearly follow-up for lifelong surveillance.[10] Lifelong surveillance (>10 years) is not uncommon. CT of the abdomen and pelvis is the

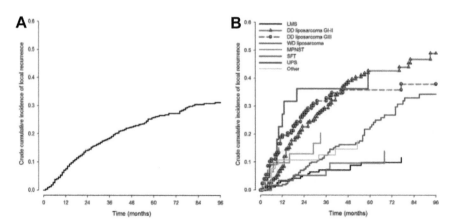

Fig. 9. (*A*) Crude cumulative incidence of local recurrence for the whole series; (*B*) Crude cumulative incidence of local recurrence by histologic subtype. DD, dedifferentiated; GI-III, grades I-III; LMS, leiomyosarcoma; MPNST, malignant peripheral nerve sheath tumor; SFT, solitary fibrous tumor; UPS, undifferentiated pleomorphic sarcoma; WD, well-differentiated. (*From* Gronchi et al., with permission.[2])

preferred imaging modality to assess for locoregional recurrence. A CT chest without IV contrast is recommended for patients where distant metastases are possible, although a 2-view chest X-ray is acceptable for patients diagnosed with low-grade/well-differentiated RPS because the risk of distant recurrence is exceedingly low.[49] At this time, there are no randomized controlled trials evaluating the optimal surveillance strategy for RPS. However, given histology-specific patterns of recurrence, a more individualized surveillance approach, particularly for the most common histologies, is often pursued.

SUMMARY

Given that RPS consists of several different sarcoma histologies, there are notable challenges to the diagnosis, management, and surveillance of this rare disease. Involvement of an experienced multidisciplinary team at a specialized sarcoma center is key to developing a histology-specific treatment plan, which can increase the likelihood of a curative oncologic resection. Although there is limited randomized, controlled trial data on the utility of multimodality treatment strategies for RPS, there is likely a role for neoadjuvant radiation therapy and/or chemotherapy, carefully considered on a patient-by-patient basis. Similarly, surveillance strategies should be tailored to the specific RPS histology. Although significant progress has been made in recent decades, continued international cooperation and collaboration remain imperative to improve the management of RPS patients.

CLINICS CARE POINTS

- Given the heterogeneity of retroperitoneal sarcomas (RPS), careful consideration of disease histology and location is crucial, to aid in diagnosis, management, and long-term surveillance.

- For localized, primary RPS s, adjacent critical organs and vascular structures must be accounted for to ensure a wide margin of resection.

- As the management strategies for sarcomas continue to evolve, use the expertise of a multidisciplinary tumor board at specialized sarcoma referral centers.

AUTHOR CONTRIBUTIONS

(I). Conception and design: all authors
(II). Administrative support: all authors
(III). Provision of study materials or patients: not applicable
(IV). Collection and assembly of data: not applicable
(V). Data analysis and interpretation: not applicable
(VI). Article writing: all authors
(VII). Final approval of article: all authors

ETHICAL STATEMENT

The authors are accountable for all aspects of the article in ensuring that questions related to the accuracy or integrity of any part of the article are appropriately investigated and resolved.

DISCLOSURE

The authors do not have commercial or financial conflicts of interest and no additional funding sources.

REFERENCES

1. Brennan MF, Antonescu CR, Moraco N, et al. Lessons learned from the study of 10,000 patients with soft tissue sarcoma. Ann Surg 2014;260(3):416–21 [discussion: 421-2].
2. Gronchi A, Strauss DC, Miceli R, et al. Variability in patterns of recurrence after resection of primary retroperitoneal sarcoma (RPS): a report on 1007 patients from the multi-institutional collaborative RPS working group. Ann Surg 2016; 263(5):1002–9.
3. Jo VY, Fletcher CD. WHO classification of soft tissue tumours: an update based on the 2013 (4th) edition. Pathology 2014;46(2):95–104.
4. Linehan DC, Lewis JJ, Leung D, et al. Influence of biologic factors and anatomic site in completely resected liposarcoma. J Clin Oncol 2000;18(8):1637–43.
5. Tan MC, Brennan MF, Kuk D, et al. Histology-based classification predicts pattern of recurrence and improves risk stratification in primary retroperitoneal sarcoma. Ann Surg 2016;263(3):593–600.
6. Gronchi A, Miceli R, Allard MA, et al. Personalizing the approach to retroperitoneal soft tissue sarcoma: histology-specific patterns of failure and postrelapse outcome after primary extended resection. Ann Surg Oncol 2015;22(5):1447–54.
7. Ronchi A, Cozzolino I, Zito Marino F, et al. Extrapleural solitary fibrous tumor: a distinct entity from pleural solitary fibrous tumor. An update on clinical, molecular and diagnostic features. Ann Diagn Pathol 2018;34:142–50.
8. Stoeckle E, Coindre JM, Bonvalot S, et al. Prognostic factors in retroperitoneal sarcoma: a multivariate analysis of a series of 165 patients of the French Cancer Center Federation Sarcoma Group. Cancer 2001;92(2):359–68.
9. Billingsley KG, Burt ME, Jara E, et al. Pulmonary metastases from soft tissue sarcoma: analysis of patterns of diseases and postmetastasis survival. Ann Surg 1999;229(5):602–10 [discussion: 610-2].
10. Network NCC. Soft tissue sarcoma. Available at: https://www.nccn.org/professionals/physician_gls/pdf/sarcoma.pdf. Accessed May 26, 2021.
11. Almond LM, Tirotta F, Tattersall H, et al. Diagnostic accuracy of percutaneous biopsy in retroperitoneal sarcoma. Br J Surg 2019;106(4):395–403.
12. Berger-Richardson D, Burtenshaw SM, Ibrahim AM, et al. Early and late complications of percutaneous core needle biopsy of retroperitoneal tumors at two tertiary sarcoma centers. Ann Surg Oncol 2019;26(13):4692–8.
13. Van Houdt WJ, Schrijver AM, Cohen-Hallaleh RB, et al. Needle tract seeding following core biopsies in retroperitoneal sarcoma. Eur J Surg Oncol 2017; 43(9):1740–5.
14. Berger-Richardson D, Swallow CJ. Needle tract seeding after percutaneous biopsy of sarcoma: Risk/benefit considerations. Cancer 2017;123(4):560–7.
15. Amin MB, Greene FL, Edge SB, et al. The eighth edition AJCC cancer staging manual: continuing to build a bridge from a population-based to a more "personalized" approach to cancer staging. CA Cancer J Clin 2017;67(2):93–9.
16. Gronchi A, Miceli R, Shurell E, et al. Outcome prediction in primary resected retroperitoneal soft tissue sarcoma: histology-specific overall survival and disease-free survival nomograms built on major sarcoma center data sets. J Clin Oncol 2013;31(13):1649–55.

17. Management of primary retroperitoneal sarcoma (RPS) in the adult: a consensus approach from the Trans-Atlantic RPS Working Group. Ann Surg Oncol 2015; 22(1):256–63.
18. Casali PG, Abecassis N, Aro HT, et al. Soft tissue and visceral sarcomas: ESMO-EURACAN Clinical Practice Guidelines for diagnosis, treatment and follow-up. Ann Oncol 2018;29(Suppl 4):iv51–67.
19. Raut CP, Bonvalot S, Gronchi A. A call to action: Why sarcoma surgery needs to be centralized. Cancer 2018;124(23):4452–4.
20. Blay JY, Honoré C, Stoeckle E, et al. Surgery in reference centers improves survival of sarcoma patients: a nationwide study. Ann Oncol 2019;30(7):1143–53.
21. Keung EZ, Chiang YJ, Cormier JN, et al. Treatment at low-volume hospitals is associated with reduced short-term and long-term outcomes for patients with retroperitoneal sarcoma. Cancer 2018;124(23):4495–503.
22. Keung EZ, Hornick JL, Bertagnolli MM, et al. Predictors of outcomes in patients with primary retroperitoneal dedifferentiated liposarcoma undergoing surgery. J Am Coll Surg 2014;218(2):206–17.
23. Gyorki DE, Brennan MF. Management of recurrent retroperitoneal sarcoma. J Surg Oncol 2014;109(1):53–9.
24. Callegaro D, Raut CP, Ng D, et al. Has the outcome for patients who undergo resection of primary retroperitoneal sarcoma changed over time? A study of time trends during the past 15 years. Ann Surg Oncol 2021;28(3):1700–9.
25. Stahl JM, Corso CD, Park HS, et al. The effect of microscopic margin status on survival in adult retroperitoneal soft tissue sarcomas. Eur J Surg Oncol 2017; 43(1):168–74.
26. Jaques DP, Coit DG, Hajdu SI, et al. Management of primary and recurrent soft-tissue sarcoma of the retroperitoneum. Ann Surg 1990;212(1):51–9.
27. Ng D, Swallow CJ. Decision-making for palliative versus curative intent treatment of retroperitoneal sarcoma (RPS). Chin Clin Oncol 2018;7(4):40.
28. Gronchi A, Lo Vullo S, Fiore M, et al. Aggressive surgical policies in a retrospectively reviewed single-institution case series of retroperitoneal soft tissue sarcoma patients. J Clin Oncol 2009;27(1):24–30.
29. Bonvalot S, Rivoire M, Castaing M, et al. Primary retroperitoneal sarcomas: a multivariate analysis of surgical factors associated with local control. J Clin Oncol 2009;27(1):31–7.
30. Tzanis D, Bouhadiba T, Gaignard E, et al. Major vascular resections in retroperitoneal sarcoma. J Surg Oncol 2018;117(1):42–7.
31. Gamboa AC, Gronchi A, Cardona K. Soft-tissue sarcoma in adults: an update on the current state of histiotype-specific management in an era of personalized medicine. CA Cancer J Clin 2020;70(3):200–29.
32. Gronchi A, Miceli R, Colombo C, et al. Frontline extended surgery is associated with improved survival in retroperitoneal low- to intermediate-grade soft tissue sarcomas. Ann Oncol 2012;23(4):1067–73.
33. O'Sullivan B, Davis AM, Turcotte R, et al. Preoperative versus postoperative radiotherapy in soft-tissue sarcoma of the limbs: a randomised trial. Lancet 2002;359(9325):2235–41.
34. Gingrich AA, Bateni SB, Monjazeb AM, et al. Neoadjuvant radiotherapy is associated with r0 resection and improved survival for patients with extremity soft tissue sarcoma undergoing surgery: a national cancer database analysis. Ann Surg Oncol 2017;24(11):3252–63.

35. Davis AM, O'Sullivan B, Turcotte R, et al. Late radiation morbidity following randomization to preoperative versus postoperative radiotherapy in extremity soft tissue sarcoma. Radiother Oncol 2005;75(1):48–53.
36. Nussbaum DP, Rushing CN, Lane WO, et al. Preoperative or postoperative radiotherapy versus surgery alone for retroperitoneal sarcoma: a case-control, propensity score-matched analysis of a nationwide clinical oncology database. Lancet Oncol 2016;17(7):966–75.
37. Bonvalot S, Gronchi A, Le Péchoux C, et al. Preoperative radiotherapy plus surgery versus surgery alone for patients with primary retroperitoneal sarcoma (EORTC-62092: STRASS): a multicentre, open-label, randomised, phase 3 trial. Lancet Oncol 2020;21(10):1366–77.
38. McBride SM, Raut CP, Lapidus M, et al. Locoregional recurrence after preoperative radiation therapy for retroperitoneal sarcoma: adverse impact of multifocal disease and potential implications of dose escalation. Ann Surg Oncol 2013; 20(7):2140–7.
39. Radaelli S, Stacchiotti S, Casali PG, et al. Emerging therapies for adult soft tissue sarcoma. Expert Rev Anticancer Ther 2014;14(6):689–704.
40. Adjuvant chemotherapy for localised resectable soft-tissue sarcoma of adults: meta-analysis of individual data. Sarcoma Meta-analysis Collaboration. Lancet 1997;350(9092):1647–54.
41. Issels RD, Lindner LH, Verweij J, et al. Effect of Neoadjuvant Chemotherapy Plus Regional Hyperthermia on Long-term Outcomes Among Patients With Localized High-Risk Soft Tissue Sarcoma: The EORTC 62961-ESHO 95 Randomized Clinical Trial. JAMA Oncol 2018;4(4):483–92.
42. Meric F, Milas M, Hunt KK, et al. Impact of neoadjuvant chemotherapy on postoperative morbidity in soft tissue sarcomas. J Clin Oncol 2000;18(19):3378–83.
43. Miura JT, Charlson J, Gamblin TC, et al. Impact of chemotherapy on survival in surgically resected retroperitoneal sarcoma. Eur J Surg Oncol 2015;41(10): 1386–92.
44. Singer S, Antonescu CR, Riedel E, et al. Histologic subtype and margin of resection predict pattern of recurrence and survival for retroperitoneal liposarcoma. Ann Surg 2003;238(3):358–71.
45. Chouliaras K, Senehi R, Ethun CG, et al. Recurrence patterns after resection of retroperitoneal sarcomas: an eight-institution study from the US Sarcoma Collaborative. J Surg Oncol 2019;120(3):340–7.
46. Lewis JJ, Leung D, Woodruff JM, et al. Retroperitoneal soft-tissue sarcoma: analysis of 500 patients treated and followed at a single institution. Ann Surg 1998; 228(3):355–65.
47. MacNeill AJ, Miceli R, Strauss DC, et al. Post-relapse outcomes after primary extended resection of retroperitoneal sarcoma: a report from the Trans-Atlantic RPS Working Group. Cancer 2017;123(11):1971–8.
48. Bagaria SP, Gabriel E, Mann GN. Multiply recurrent retroperitoneal liposarcoma. J Surg Oncol 2018;117(1):62–8.
49. Zaidi MY, Canter R, Cardona K. Post-operative surveillance in retroperitoneal soft tissue sarcoma: The importance of tumor histology in guiding strategy. J Surg Oncol 2018;117(1):99–104.
50. Turgeon MK, Cardona K. Soft tissue tumors of the abdomen and retroperitoneum. Surg Clin North Am 2020;100(3):649–67.

Sarcoma Pulmonary Metastatic Disease

Still a Chance for Cure

Mark Hennon, MD[a,b,*]

KEYWORDS

- Soft tissue sarcoma • Pulmonary metastases • Metastasectomy
- Video-assisted thoracoscopic surgery (VATS) • Pulmonary resection

KEY POINTS

- Pulmonary metastasectomy in carefully selected patients improves long term survival.
- Systemic therapy options, though increasing, are still limited and have limited effectiveness.
- Minimally invasive approaches are safe, and do not compromise outcomes.
- Expanding technology is improving the surgeon's ability to identify small lung nodules with minimally invasive approaches.

INTRODUCTION

Sarcomas are uncommon, accounting for 1% of all cancers. Approximately 13,190 new cases (7590 men, 5600 women) are expected in the United States in 2022 with 5130 deaths attributed to metastatic sarcoma.[1] Sarcomas represent a heterogenous group of tumors and can behave with varying degrees of aggressiveness. The most common histologic types include undifferentiated pleomorphic sarcoma, liposarcoma, and leiomyosarcoma. Given the rare and heterogeneous nature, determining an effective treatment for the patient with sarcoma can be challenging and is best achieved in a multidisciplinary setting.

Approximately 20% to 50% of patients with sarcoma will develop hematogenous metastases to the lungs. Tumors with high-grade pathology have an increased rate of systemic metastasis (>50%) as compared with 10% for tumors with low-grade pathology.[2] Osteosarcoma represents the histologic subtype most likely to metastasize to the lung, followed by synovial sarcoma and liposarcoma.[3] Pulmonary metastatic sarcoma negatively impacts prognosis and reduces the overall 5-year survival of

Funded by: NIHEFD.
[a] Department of Thoracic Surgery, Roswell Park Comprehensive Cancer Center, Elm and Carlton Streets, Buffalo, NY 14263, USA; [b] Department of Surgery, Jacobs School of Medicine, State University of New York at Buffalo, 100 High Street, Buffalo, NY 14203, USA
* Corresponding author. Department of Thoracic Surgery, Roswell Park Comprehensive Cancer Center, Elm and Carlton Streets, Buffalo, NY 14263.
E-mail address: mark.hennon@roswellpark.org

Surg Clin N Am 102 (2022) 615–624
https://doi.org/10.1016/j.suc.2022.05.001
0039-6109/22/Published by Elsevier Inc.

patients from approximately 65% to 15% to 52%.[3-6] For patients who develop metastatic disease, systemic therapy is frequently used, but, unfortunately, has limited impact on improving survival. Recent advances in the understanding of soft tissue sarcoma tumor biology at the molecular level have increased systemic therapy options to include immunotherapies and occasionally targeted therapies.[7,8] Despite some improvements in systemic therapy, surgical resection of pulmonary metastases is often the preferred treatment option for patients who are appropriate surgical candidates, as the clearance of metastatic disease with surgical resection has been shown to be cost-effective and, more importantly, can improve the chances for long-term survival.[3-6,9-14]

When considering surgical resection for patients with pulmonary sarcoma metastases, the primary objectives are to minimize morbidity and maximize long-term survival. This can be challenging, and the decision on whether to offer surgery is made on an individualized basis. Factors, such as tumor histology (leiomyosarcoma has been shown in series to be a favorable prognostic indicator), number of metastases, location of the metastases, time from primary tumor treatment to development of pulmonary metastases, as well as individual patient comorbidities, can impact both the short-term and the long-term outcomes for patients undergoing pulmonary metastasectomy. Minimally invasive approaches to pulmonary resection for primary lung tumors have been shown to reduce short-term morbidity and expand operative treatment options for medically frail patients; this same rationale applies to patients undergoing metastasectomy for sarcoma metastases as well.[15,16] Initial concerns regarding compromised long-term oncologic outcomes with minimally invasive approaches were largely due to the potential for missed/unrecognized lung lesions resulting from the limited ability for intraoperative lung palpation. A universal approach to the patient with pulmonary metastatic sarcoma is not feasible. However, with careful patient selection, long-term survival can be achieved.

HISTORICAL CONSIDERATIONS

- Effective systemic therapies for metastatic sarcoma, although increasing in number, are still limited.
- Complete surgical resection of pulmonary disease with negative margins improves long-term survival.
- Criteria for patient selection have changed little over time, although minimally invasive approaches reduce perioperative morbidity and have expanded surgical options.

Historically, options for managing metastatic disease to the lungs in patients with soft tissue sarcoma have been limited. Effective systemic therapies for improving long-term survival are lacking. The morbidity and mortality associated with metastasectomy, although relatively low, were not insignificant with traditional open surgical approaches. The first pulmonary metastasectomy was described in the late 1800s by Weinlechner.[17] It was not until 1947 that a survival benefit for patients with sarcoma undergoing pulmonary metastasectomy was reported.[18] Selection criteria described at that time for appropriate surgical candidates remain valid to this day. The classical tenets for considering pulmonary metastasectomy include a controlled primary site without local recurrence, adequate disease-free interval (the longer the better), absence of extrathoracic disease, and disease that can be resected in its entirety with negative margins. Other criteria to consider include the cardiopulmonary reserve of the patient and tumor histology (leiomyosarcoma histology has better long-term outcomes vs undifferentiated pleomorphic sarcoma/malignant fibrous histiosarcoma).

The era of minimally invasive thoracic surgery has allowed for some exceptions to the classical selection criteria in carefully selected scenarios. For example, for patients presenting with a synchronous, isolated, peripherally located lung metastasis in the setting of a primary sarcoma that will require an extensive resection and complex reconstruction, removing the solitary lung met thoracoscopically with minimal risk of perioperative morbidity may be reasonable before treating the primary tumor.

Historical series examining the impact of pulmonary metastasectomy for sarcoma are entirely retrospective. There are no randomized controlled trials providing formal evidence for the effectiveness of pulmonary metastasectomy and are unlikely to ever be performed given the ethical concerns over withholding potentially curative treatment in a randomized setting. Retrospective series showing long-term survival benefit are numerous, but have inherent limitations, notably selection bias.[3–6,9–14,19–26] In one of the largest ever published single-institution retrospective analyses (of a prospectively maintained database) involving more than 800 patients, primary tumor histologic subtype, size, number of pulmonary metastases, disease-free interval, and selection for minimally invasive resection were all associated with increased survival.[27] **Table 1** includes a summary of more recent retrospective series demonstrating a survival benefit for pulmonary metastasectomy for soft tissue sarcoma.

SURGICAL CONSIDERATIONS FOR PULMONARY METASTASECTOMY
Overall Objectives

- Resect disease while minimizing morbidity
- Spare lung parenchyma
- Achieve negative margins
- Minimally invasive approaches by video-assisted thoracoscopic surgery (VATS) are acceptable

Pulmonary metastasectomy for curative intent involves resecting all metastatic disease with negative margins, while minimizing surgical morbidity. Surgical morbidity following lung resection is potentially influenced by multiple factors. The extent of total lung parenchyma resected as well as the surgical approach can impact outcomes. Given the desire to minimize morbidity and preserve lung function, pulmonary wedge resection with negative margins is frequently the surgical plan. In specific instances, anatomic resection with lobectomy may be necessary based on lesion size or location and is not unreasonable to consider.

Wedge Resection

Pulmonary wedge resection of all lung nodules with negative parenchymal margins is the objective in most clinical scenarios. For lung lesions located on the periphery of the lung, minimally invasive approaches allow for metastasectomy with minimal morbidity.

Anatomic Resection

Segmentectomy, lobectomy, and pneumonectomy

For centrally located lung lesions, wedge resection may not be feasible. In this situation, anatomic lung resection is not contraindicated. In a large retrospective series focusing only on perioperative outcomes, 33/327 patients underwent lobectomy for pulmonary sarcoma metastases with no perioperative mortality and only 2.8% risk for major morbidity.[28] When possible, a parenchymal sparing approach with segmentectomy should be considered, can be performed minimally invasively without compromising oncologic principles, and has been well described.[29] Long-term survival is possible with pneumonectomy, although not without the potential for increased morbidity and

Table 1
Studies evaluating long-term outcomes for patients undergoing pulmonary metastasectomy for soft tissue sarcoma

Authors, y	Journal	Country	Patients	Survival (%)[a]	VATS/Open	Summary
Chen et al,[24] 2009	Eur J Surg Oncol	Japan	23	43	N/A	Repeat metastasectomy provided favorable response
Smith et al,[6] 2009	Eur J Surg Oncol	US	94	18	Open	Mean DFI 25 mo, 74 with R0 resection, DFI and R0 associated with improved OS
Burt et al,[31] 2011	Ann Thorac Surg	US	82	52/32	Both	Subset of leiomyosarcoma, repeat PM, had OS 70 vs 24 mo for nonleiomyosarcoma histology
Reza et al,[23] 2014	J Thorac Cardiovascular Surg	US	145	42	Both	Median survival 35 mo, minimally invasive approach not associated with a decrease in survival
Dossett et al,[20] 2015	J Surg Oncol	US	120	44	Both	2000–2012, median overall survival 48 mo, synchronous metastases, older age, and number of lesions were associated with decreased survival
Lin et al,[22] 2015	J Thorac Cardiovasc Surg	US	155	34.8	Both	Identified factors associated with poor survival, age >45 y, DFS <1 y, thoracotomy, synchronous disease, location and histology, and lobectomy
Giuliano et al,[21] 2016	Thorac Cardiovasc Surg	US	53	28.3	Both	1989–2013, median overall survival 59.9 mo, 10-y survival 13.3%
Okiror et al,[5] 2016	Thorac Cardiovascular Surg	United Kingdom	80	N/A	Both	2007–2014, median OS 25.5 mo. Recurrence of metastases decreased survival
Chudgar et al,[27] 2017	J Thorac Cardiovascular Surg	US	803	34	Both	MIS associated with improved long-term survival
Cariboni et al,[11] 2019	Am J Clin Oncol	Italy	154	36.5	Both	1997–2015, male sex, bilateral metastasis, and histology poor prognostic indicators based on multivariable analyses. 35.4 mo median survival
Dudek et al,[13] 2019	J Thorac Dis	Germany	33	40.4	Both	No perioperative deaths, median interval between primary tumor and PM 16 mo, R0 in 93.9% patients
Yamamoto et al,[25] 2019	Int J Clin Oncol	Japan	44	60	Both	Tumor size, DFI, and R0 resection associated with improved survival, surgical approach did not impact outcomes
Shimizu et al,[26] 2020	Mol Clin Oncol.	Japan	22	53	VATS	34 total patients, no survivors beyond 3 y for nonsurgical group (n = 12)
Gusho et al,[12] 2021	Interact Cardiovasc Thorac Surg	US	565	31.2	N/A	SEER Database review 2010–2015, propensity matched, DFS 32 mo with PM, 20 without PM

mortality. This was demonstrated by the International Registry of Lung Metastases, whereby 171/5206 patients who underwent pneumonectomy had a 5-year overall survival of 20% when surgery resulted in complete resection. Perioperative mortality was 4%. Patients with sarcoma with a negative margin resection had a 5-year overall survival of 30%.[30]

Reresection

Approximately 50% of patients who undergo pulmonary metastasectomy will develop recurrent disease with some reports noting recurrence rates as high as 70%. Long-term survival can still be achieved with repeat pulmonary metastasectomy if feasible with reduced morbidity, especially in patients initially resected by minimally invasive approaches. For patients previously resected by thoracotomy or sternotomy, an open approach is likely necessary, but should be determined in consultation with a thoracic surgeon participating in a multidisciplinary setting.[31–33]

Preoperative Considerations

In addition to the previously described oncologic criteria to consider when evaluating for possible pulmonary metastasectomy, a standard cardiopulmonary evaluation is necessary to assess for the potential morbidity of the proposed surgery. Pulmonary function testing, cardiac risk stratification, and more recently, frailty testing should all be obtained as part of the surgical evaluation. Patients requiring pulmonary metastasectomy for sarcoma often do not have chronic obstructive pulmonary disease or significant cardiopulmonary risk factors attributed to patients undergoing lung resection for primary tumors of the lung.

Surgical Approach

- Traditionally performed by open approaches
- As minimally invasive techniques for lung resection evolved, they were also used for pulmonary metastasectomy
- Long-term oncologic survival concerns with minimally invasive approaches due to missed low-volume pulmonary metastatic disease at the time of surgery and port site implants are largely unfounded

Open Approaches

Traditionally, surgical resection of sarcoma pulmonary metastases was performed via a thoracotomy if the lesions were unilateral. For patients with bilateral pulmonary metastases, complete clearance of disease can be achieved through bilateral pulmonary wedge resections via a median sternotomy or bilateral anterolateral thoracotomies with transsternal extension (clamshell approach). Although open approaches potentially incur significant perioperative morbidity, long-term survival outcomes for patients who underwent pulmonary metastasectomy via open approaches continue to serve as the standard for comparison to minimally invasive techniques. Open approaches allow for bimanual palpation of the lungs, identifying up to 25% additional nodules as compared with what was noted on the preoperative staging computed tomography (CT).[34]

Minimally Invasive Approaches

Video-assisted thoracoscopic surgery, robotic-assisted thoracoscopic surgery

With the advent of low-profile viewing cameras and video systems that allow for high-resolution viewing of the thorax, minimally invasive approaches to lung resection have been described for decades, dating back to the 1980s.[35] Arguments supporting the potential benefits of a VATS approach for pulmonary metastasectomy have been made for more than 20 years.[36] Although initially controversial owing to concerns over their ability to achieve comparable outcomes for long-term overall survival, it is now accepted that minimally invasive approaches to pulmonary metastasectomy do not compromise long-term outcomes. Bimanual palpation is not feasible with VATS (although finger palpation is possible), and no tactile palpation is used with robotic approaches. Studies have demonstrated that intraoperative bimanual palpation will identify previously unrecognized nodules in 20% to 25% of cases.[34] Consequently, VATS is associated with increased recurrence rates, likely attributable to unrecognized low-volume metastatic disease. This known decreased sensitivity of VATS for the intraoperative detection of previously unrecognized metastatic nodules has understandably led to concerns regarding the impact on long-term survival. Interestingly, a large amount of retrospective data (subject to selection bias) has shown no impact on long-term outcomes for patients undergoing pulmonary metastasectomy via minimally invasive approaches. The increased ability to proceed with re-resection for unrecognized disease with less morbidity following minimally invasive approaches likely accounts for these findings.

Techniques for improving intraoperative metastasis identification

- Given the limited ability for palpation with minimally invasive approaches to lung resection, improved technology has allowed for identification of nonpalpable metastatic nodules intraoperatively.
- These techniques are applicable to pulmonary metastasectomy for sarcoma.
- Additional studies are needed to verify the effectiveness.
- Metastatic nodules requiring this degree of intraoperative assessment for identification may benefit from an additional period of radiographic surveillance.

Difficulty with intraoperative identification of small, subcentimeter pulmonary nodules is not limited to pulmonary metastasectomy. Widespread use of CT imaging for other indications, such as lung cancer screening, has led to an increase in the identification of subcentimeter, asymptomatic pulmonary nodules. Techniques and technology that have been developed over time for the intraoperative identification of nonpalpable, subcentimeter nodules can also be used for localizing sarcoma metastases. Small, presumed pulmonary metastases located deep to the pleural surface may be challenging to identify intraoperatively with minimally invasive approaches that limit manual palpation. These techniques and technology, although potentially helpful, should be considered only in a multidisciplinary setting, as the option of continued radiographic surveillance may be preferable based on multiple criteria, including tissue histology, location, and number of lesions. For example, a 5-mm nodule noted on a surveillance CT scan of the chest in the setting of a patient treated for a low-grade sarcoma may be better served with continued observation.

Percutaneous Needle Localization

Preoperative nodule localization, predominantly performed with the aid of CT guidance in either the operating room or the interventional radiology suite immediately before the planned surgical procedure can aid the surgeon in finding a nonpalpable nodule. In addition to more traditional inert methylene blue dye injection/staining, a transpleural hookwire, microcoils, or other fiducials can be used.[37] Needle localization performed in the operating room immediately before surgery using electromagnetic guidance and CT coregistration to virtually guide needle localization or methylene blue dye injection is now being used as well (SPiN System; Veran

Medical Technologies, St. Louis, MO, USA). Studies examining the impact of these techniques on long-term outcomes are lacking. Therefore, a decision on whether to proceed with pulmonary metastasectomy for lung lesions requiring localization techniques should only be made in the setting of a multidisciplinary tumor board.

Alternatives to Surgical Resection

For patients that are not appropriate surgical candidates, especially those with oligometastatic or oligoprogressive disease, stereotactic body radiation treatment and/or ablative therapies are options for consideration.[38–41]

SUMMARY

- The management of sarcoma pulmonary metastatic disease can be challenging, often requires multiple treatment modalities, and is best planned in a multidisciplinary setting.
- Systemic therapy options, although increasing, are still limited for improving long-term survival.
- Despite a lack of evidence from randomized controlled trials, pulmonary metastasectomy in carefully selected patients has been shown to improve long-term survival, even when repeat metastasectomy is necessary, and may also be cost-effective.
- Minimally invasive approaches with VATS are safe and have not been shown to compromise long-term outcomes.
- New technologies are improving the surgeon's ability to identify small lung nodules with minimally invasive approaches.
- In the future, using the resected metastatic tissue for analysis at the molecular/genetic level for systemic treatment planning may ultimately prove to be the most valuable aspect of pulmonary metastasectomy.[7,8]

CLINICS CARE POINTS

- Pulmonary metastasectomy for patients with soft tissue sarcoma in carefully selected patients improves long term survival.

- Minimally invasive approaches are safe, and do not compromise long term oncologic outcomes.

DISCLOSURE

The author has nothing to disclose.

REFERENCES

1. Siegel RL, Miller KD, Fuchs HE, et al. Cancer statistics, 2022. CA Cancer J Clin 2022. https://doi.org/10.3322/caac.21708.
2. Coindre JM, Terrier P, Guillo L, et al. Predictive value of grade for metastasis development in the main histologic types of adult soft tissue sarcoma: a study of 1240 patients from French Federation of Cancer Centers Sarcoma Group. Cancer 2001;91(10):1914–26.

3. Billingsley KG, Burt ME, Jara E, et al. Pulmonary metastases from soft tissue sarcoma: analysis of patterns of diseases and postmetastases survival. Ann Surg 1999;229(5):602–10.

4. Predina JD, Puc MM, Bergey MR, et al. Improved survival after pulmonary metastasectomy for soft tissue sarcoma. J Thorac Oncol 2011;6:913–9.

5. Okiror L, Peleki A, Moffat D, et al. Survival following Pulmonary Metastasectomy for Sarcoma. Thorac Cardiovasc Surg 2016;64(2):146–9.

6. Smith R, Pak Y, Kraybill W, et al. Factors associated actual long-term survival after pulmonary metastasectomy. Eur J Surg Oncol 2009;35:356–61.

7. Klemen ND, Kelly CM, Bartlett EK. The emerging role of immunotherapy for the treatment of sarcoma. J Surg Oncol 2021;123(3):730–8.

8. Ayodele O, Razak ARA. Immunotherapy in soft-tissue sarcoma. Curr Oncol 2020; 27(Suppl 1):17–23.

9. Pastorino U, Buyse M, Friedel G, et al, International Registry of Lung Metastases. Long-term results of lung metastasectomy: prognostic analyses based on 5206 cases. J Thorac Cardiovasc Surg 1997;113(1):37–49.

10. Smith R, Demmy TL. Pulmonary metastasectomy for soft tissue sarcoma. Surg Oncol Clin N Am 2012;21:269–86.

11. Cariboni U, De Sanctis R, Giaretta M, et al. Survival Outcome and Prognostic Factors After Pulmonary Metastasectomy in Sarcoma Patients: A 18-Year Experience at a Single High-volume Referral Center. Am J Clin Oncol 2019;42(1):6–11.

12. Gusho CA, Seder CW, Lopez-Hisijos N, et al. Pulmonary metastasectomy in bone and soft tissue sarcoma with metastasis to the lung. Interact Cardiovasc Thorac Surg 2021;33(6):879–84.

13. Dudek W, Schreiner W, Mykoliuk I, et al. Pulmonary metastasectomy for sarcoma-survival and prognostic analysis. J Thorac Dis 2019;11(8):3369–76.

14. Porter GA, Cantor SB, Walsh GL, et al. Cost-effectiveness of pulmonary resection and systemic chemotherapy in the management of metastatic soft tissue sarcoma: a combined analysis from the University of Texas M. D. Anderson and Memorial Sloan-Kettering Cancer Centers. J Thorac Cardiovasc Surg 2004;127(5):1366–72.

15. Landreneau RJ, Wiechmann RJ, Hazelrigg SR, et al. Effect of minimally invasive thoracic surgical approaches on acute and chronic postoperative pain. Chest Surg Clin N Am 1998;8(4):891–906.

16. Demmy TL, Curtis JJ. Minimally invasive lobectomy directed toward frail and high-risk patients: a case-control study. Ann Thorac Surg 1999;68(1):194–200.

17. Weinlechner J. Tumoren an der brustwand und deren behnadlung resection der rippeneroffnung der brusthohle und partielle entfernungder lunge. Weiner Med Wrsh 1882;32:589–91.

18. Alexander J, Haight C. Pulmonary resection for solitary metastatic sarcoma and carcinomas. Surg Gynecol Obst 1947;85(2):129–46.

19. Blackmon SH, Shah N, Roth JA, et al. Resection of pulmonary and extrapulmonary sarcomatous metastases is associated with long-term survival. Ann Thorac Surg 2009;88(3):877–84 [discussion: 884–5].

20. Dossett LA, Toloza EM, Fontaine J, et al. Outcomes and clinical predictors of improved survival in a patients undergoing pulmonary metastasectomy for sarcoma. J Surg Oncol 2015;112(1):103–6.

21. Giuliano K, Sachs T, Montgomery E, et al. Survival Following Lung Metastasectomy in Soft Tissue Sarcomas. Thorac Cardiovasc Surg 2016;64(2):150–8.

22. Lin AY, Kotova S, Yanagawa J, et al. Risk stratification of patients undergoing pulmonary metastasectomy for soft tissue and bone sarcomas. J Thorac Cardiovasc Surg 2015;149(1):85–92.
23. Reza J, Sammann A, Jin C, et al. Aggressive and minimally invasive surgery for pulmonary metastasis of sarcoma. J Thorac Cardiovasc Surg 2014;147(4): 1193–200 [discussion: 1200–1].
24. Chen F, Fujinaga T, Sato K, et al. Significance of tumor recurrence before pulmonary metastasis in pulmonary metastasectomy for soft tissue sarcoma. Eur J Surg Oncol 2009;35(6):660–5.
25. Yamamoto Y, Kanzaki R, Kanou T, et al. Long-term outcomes and prognostic factors of pulmonary metastasectomy for osteosarcoma and soft tissue sarcoma. Int J Clin Oncol 2019;24(7):863–70.
26. Shimizu J, Emori M, Murahashi Y, et al. Pulmonary metastasectomy is associated with prolonged survival among patients with bone and soft tissue sarcoma. Mol Clin Oncol 2020;12(5):429–34.
27. Chudgar NP, Brennan MF, Munhoz RR, et al. Pulmonary metastasectomy with therapeutic intent for soft-tissue sarcoma. J Thorac Cardiovasc Surg 2017; 154(1):319–30.e1.
28. Gafencu DA, Welter S, Cheufou DH, et al. Pulmonary metastasectomy for sarcoma-Essen experience. J Thorac Dis 2017;9(Suppl 12):S1278–81.
29. Berry MF. Role of segmentectomy for pulmonary metastases. Ann Cardiothorac Surg 2014;3(2):176–82.
30. Koong HN, Pastorino U, Ginsberg RJ. Is there a role for pneumonectomy in pulmonary metastases? International Registry of Lung Metastases. Ann Thorac Surg 1999;68(6):2039–43.
31. Burt BM, Ocejo S, Mery CM, et al. Repeated and aggressive pulmonary resections for leiomyosarcoma metastases extends survival. Ann Thorac Surg 2011; 92(4):1202–7.
32. Chudgar NP, Brennan MF, Tan KS, et al. Is Repeat Pulmonary Metastasectomy Indicated for Soft Tissue Sarcoma? Ann Thorac Surg 2017;104(6):1837–45.
33. Chen F, Miyahara R, Bando T, et al. Repeat resection of pulmonary metastasis is beneficial for patients with osteosarcoma of the extremities. Interact Cardiovasc Thorac Surg 2009;9(4):649–53.
34. Cerfolio RJ, Bryant AS, McCarty TP, et al. A prospective study to determine the incidence of non-imaged malignant pulmonary nodule in patients who undergo metastasectomy by thoracotomy with lung palpation. Ann Thorac Surg 2011; 91:1696–701.
35. Loddenkemper R, Mathur PN, Lee P, et al. History and clinical use of thorascopy/ pleuroscopy in respiratory medicine. Breathe 2011;8:145–55.
36. Sonett JR. Pulmonary metastases: biologic and historical justification for VATS. Eur J Cardiothorac Surg 1999;16(Suppl 1). S13–S16.
37. Finley RJ, Mayo JR, Grant K, et al. Preoperative computed tomography-guided microcoil localization of small peripheral pulmonary nodules: a prospective randomized controlled trial. J Thorac Cardiovasc Surg 2015;149(1):26–31.
38. Greto D, Loi M, Stocchi G, et al. Stereotactic Body Radiotherapy in Oligomestatic/ Oligoprogressive Sarcoma: Safety and Effectiveness Beyond Intrinsic Radiosensitivity. Cancer J 2021;27(6):423–7.
39. Benkhaled S, Mané M, Jungels C, et al. Successful treatment of synchronous chemoresistant pulmonary metastasis from pleomorphic rhabdomyosarcoma with stereotaxic body radiation therapy: A case report and a review of the literature. Cancer Treat Res Commun 2021;26:100282.

40. Farooqi A, Mitra D, Guadagnolo BA, et al. The Evolving Role of Radiation Therapy in Patients with Metastatic Soft Tissue Sarcoma. Curr Oncol Rep 2020;22(8):79.
41. Tetta C, Carpenzano M, Algargoush ATJ, et al. Non-surgical Treatments for Lung Metastases in Patients with Soft Tissue Sarcoma: Stereotactic Body Radiation Therapy (SBRT) and Radiofrequency Ablation (RFA). Curr Med Imaging 2021; 17(2):261–75.

Gastrointestinal Stromal Tumors and the General Surgeon

Ilaria Caturegli, MD*, Chandrajit P. Raut, MD, MSc*

KEYWORDS

- Gastrointestinal stromal tumor • Sarcoma • Surgery • Adjuvant therapy
- Neoadjuvant therapy • Metastases • GIST

KEY POINTS

- Surgery is recommended for subclinical (less than 2 cm and asymptomatic) intestinal GISTs and gastric GISTs with high-risk features (include irregular border, cystic spaces, ulceration, echogenic foci, heterogeneity, and progression during follow-up).
- Clinically relevant (greater than 2 cm or symptomatic) and localized GISTs warrant oncologic resection followed by adjuvant targeted therapy with imatinib for lesions with intermediate to high recurrence risk (eg, large tumor size, high mitotic rate, and tumor site) administered for at least 3 years.
- Neoadjuvant therapy should be considered for at least 6 months before oncologic resection in lesions in which tumor size reduction would decrease the morbidity of resection, increase organ preservation, or facilitate complete oncologic resection.
- Targeted therapy is the standard of care for metastatic GISTs although surgery may be an appropriate "adjuvant" treatment for patients with the responsive disease, stable disease, or limited unifocal progression.

DEMOGRAPHICS AND GENETICS

Gastrointestinal stromal tumors or GISTs are mesenchymal or subepthelial neoplasms originating from the interstitial cells of Cajal or intestinal pacemaker cells. They make up approximately 0.1% to 3% of primary gastrointestinal malignancies with an overall incidence of 7 to 15 per million persons per year.[1,2] They present at a mean age of 60 to 65 years and arise anywhere along the gastrointestinal tract.[2,3] Most originate in the stomach (approximately 60%), whereas the balance arises in the small intestine (35%), colon or rectum (5%), or esophagus (1%).[4]

Department of Surgery, Brigham and Women's Hospital, Center for Sarcoma and Bone Oncology, Dana-Farber Cancer Institute, Harvard Medical School, 75 Francis Street, Boston, MA 02115, USA
* Corresponding authors.
E-mail addresses: ICATUREGLI@BWH.HARVARD.EDU (I.C.); CRAUT@BWH.HARVARD.EDU (C.P.R.)

Surg Clin N Am 102 (2022) 625–636
https://doi.org/10.1016/j.suc.2022.04.005   surgical.theclinics.com
0039-6109/22/© 2022 Elsevier Inc. All rights reserved.

GISTs are classically associated with mutations in the *KIT* proto-oncogene (80%) or the similar platelet-derived growth factor alpha (*PDGFRA*) (10%). These encode receptor tyrosine kinases, and pathogenic mutations lead to ligand-independent activation resulting in cell proliferation.[5] Less commonly, pathogenic mutations may be detected in *NF1* and *SDH* genes (**Table 1**). Following these early genetic changes, subsequent mutations lead to tumor proliferation, including loss of expression of the helix-loop-helix leucine zipper transcription factor MYC-associated factor X (*MAX*), which in turn leads to inactivation of a cyclin-dependent kinase inhibitor protein, p16, and cell cycle perturbation.[6] Accumulation of additional mutations contributes to tumor progression, including in the tumor suppressor *DMD* gene encoding dystrophin.[6]

Although the majority of GISTs are sporadic, there are several clinical syndromes associated with GISTs. These include Carney triad (characterized by gastric GIST, paraganglioma, and pulmonary chondromas), Carney–Stratakis syndrome or dyad (GIST and paraganglioma), neurofibromatosis 1 (associated with multicentric GISTs), and congenital *KIT* mutation (multiple GISTs present at the early age along with pigmented skin macules and urticaria pigmentosa).[7-11]

SMALL GASTROINTESTINAL STROMAL TUMORS

Small GISTs are divided into two subcategories–mini GISTs, defined as those between 1 and 2 cm, and micro GISTs, defined as those less than 1 cm. Although the true incidence of these small tumors is not well described, in the stomach, they have been

Table 1
Gastrointestinal stromal tumor genotypes

Genotype	Relative Frequency (%)
KIT mutation	70–80
Exon 8	Rare
Exon 9 insertion AY502–503	10
Exon 11 (deletions, single-nucleotide substutions, and insertions)	67
Exon 13 K642 E	1
Exon 17 D820Y, N822 K, and Y823D	1
PDGFRA mutation	5–15
Exon 12	1
Exon 14	<1
Exon 18 D842 V	5
Exon 18 (eg, deletion IMHD 842–846)	1
KIT and PDGFRA wild type	12–15
BRAF V600 E	3
SDHA, SDHB, SDHC, SDHD	3
SDHC hypermethylation	Rare
NF1	Rare
Quadruple wild type	Rare

Patil, D. T., & Rubin, B. P. (2015). Genetics of gastrointestinal stromal tumors: a heterogeneous family of tumors. Surgical Pathology Clinics, 8(3), 515-524.

reported in 10% to 35% of pathology and autopsy studies.[12–14] These lesions are usually asymptomatic and thus diagnosed either incidentally at the time of imaging or endoscopy for evaluation of other pathologies or on pathologic examination after resection for other pathologies.[15] When identified endoscopically or radiographically, the differential diagnosis for submucosal tumors (SMTs) includes both neoplasms, such as GIST, neuroendocrine tumor, leiomyoma, schwannoma, and lipoma, as well as nonneoplastic entities, such as ectopic pancreatic tumor, duplication cyst, and isolated varices.[15]

When identified, one key imaging and diagnostic modality is endoscopic ultrasound (EUS).[15] For GISTs, this modality classically demonstrates an elastic, firm, well-demarcated, hypoechoic lesion.[16,17] EUS can prove useful in distinguishing GISTs from other SMT via characteristics such as elasticity.[18–20] If the lesion is greater than 1 cm and is suspected to be a GIST, a fine needle aspiration (FNA) or fine needle biopsy (FNB) for gastric lesions or conventional biopsy for esophageal or intestinal lesions should be performed.[18,21–23] Otherwise, periodic follow-up with interval imaging, initially at 6 months and then annually, is recommended.[24]

Small GISTs less than 2 cm in size can further be subdivided by anatomic location as this determines their natural progression and, therefore, management. In general, gastric GISTs under 2 cm in size are usually found in the muscularis propria of the upper stomach. Many follow a benign progression and commonly have little to no mitotic activity.[14,21,25] These GISTs that show "benign" behavior usually harbor different genetic mutations from clinically relevant GISTs.[14] However, they may exhibit a potential for malignancy if the following high-risk EUS features are present: irregular borders, cystic spaces, ulceration, echogenic foci, internal heterogeneity, or tumor progression during follow-up.[18,21] In contrast, sub-2 cm intestinal GISTs exhibit more mitotic activity, growth, and, therefore, potential for malignancy.[21,26,27]

The following algorithm from Nishida and colleagues[15] provides a general schema for the workup and management of small GISTs (**Fig. 1**). For gastric GISTs smaller than 2 cm and without high-risk features, serial EUS is recommended.[24] Notably, less than 5% will exhibit interval growth in 2 years.[28–30] For intestinal GISTs and gastric GISTs with high-risk features, surgery is recommended.[15,18,21] The goals of resection are a macroscopically complete resection with negative microscopic margins (R0 resection) and prevention of tumor rupture to avoid tumor seeding and intraperitoneal contamination.[3,15,18,21] For most tumors, a gastric wedge resection or segmental small bowel resection is sufficient as long as the above principles are followed.[3] Lymphadenectomy is rarely indicated. In addition, resection should be performed with care to avoid a remnant stomach deformity, which may lead to gastric malfunction.[3,18,21]

Several approaches may be appropriate for resection depending on tumor location. Resection may be performed via an open, laparoscopic, laparoscopic-assisted, robotic, laparoscopic- and endoscopic-combined approach.[31–35] The use of intraoperative endoscopy may assist in the identification of these small tumors and further delineation of appropriate surgical margins.[35–37] Secondarily, it may assist in assessing the remaining luminal space or remnant deformity as well as assure intraluminal hemostasis. Strictly endoscopic resection is not recommended for GISTs as full-thickness resection may lead to an increased risk of tumor cell seeding or gastric perforation.[18,21]

CLINICALLY RELEVANT GASTROINTESTINAL STROMAL TUMORS

Clinically relevant GISTs are defined as lesions that are greater than 2 cm or symptomatic. The estimated incidence is approximately one per 100,000 per year with an

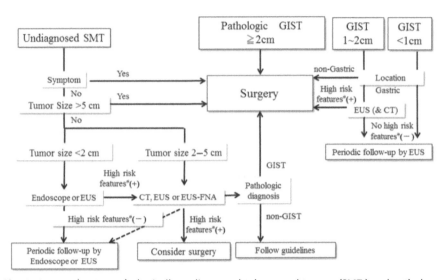

Fig. 1. Approaches to pathologically undiagnosed submucosal tumors (SMTs) and pathologically confirmed gastrointestinal stromal tumors (GISTs) are illustrated. Therapeutic approaches for pathologic GISTs are divided by size (ie, $\geq$2 cm, 1–2 cm, and <1 cm). High-risk features include irregular border, cystic spaces, ulceration, echogenic foci, heterogeneity, and progression during follow-up. CT indicates computed tomography; EUS, endoscopic ultrasonography; EUS-FNA, endoscopic ultrasonography-guided fine-needle aspiration biopsy.

overall prevalence of 5000 cases per year in the United States.[38,39] Their presentation may either be asymptomatic as an incidental finding in up to 25% of cases or be symptomatic presenting with abdominal discomfort, early satiety, bleeding, constipation, or obstruction.[40] The differential diagnosis, best elucidated after immunohistochemical staining, includes other malignant neoplastic entities, such as leiomyosarcoma, melanoma, peripheral nerve sheath tumor, inflammatory myofibroblastic tumor, and metaplastic carcinoma. Benign entities, such as leiomyoma, schwannoma, and desmoid tumors, should also be considered.[41]

The diagnostic evaluation of clinically relevant GISTs involves three components: radiographic characterization of the primary tumor, tissue diagnosis, and evaluation for metastatic disease. For characterization of the primary tumor, oral and intravenous contrast-enhanced abdominal and pelvic computed tomography (CT) is the cross-sectional modality of choice.[3] GISTs are typically characterized as a solid enhancing lesion with smooth contours; however, if necrosis or hemorrhage is present, they may appear more complex. If CT cannot be performed, magnetic resonance imaging (MRI) is an appropriate alternative and is preferred for rectal GISTs.

To obtain a tissue diagnosis, ultrasound-guided endoscopic fine-needle aspiration or biopsy with forceps is the preferred method. In contrast to percutaneous biopsy techniques, endoscopic biopsy with ultrasound permits targeted tissue sampling (increasing diagnostic yield) and decreases the hypothetical risk of tumor rupture and dissemination.[3,42] EUS-guided FNA is reported to have an 82% sensitivity and 100% specificity.[43] If biopsy is not feasible due to tumor location or if previous attempts have been nondiagnostic, laparoscopic excision may be pursued.[3] Mutational analysis of the tissue sample should be performed as this has both prognostic and therapeutic implications.

As compared to other malignancies, staging imaging for GISTs can be more limited. GISTs typically spread to other sites within the peritoneum or hematogenously the liver, so abdominal/pelvic imaging should suffice. A chest CT is not typically needed, as GISTs rarely metastasize to the lungs. A positron emission tomography (PET) scan may also be obtained on a case-by-case basis, for example, to gauge the treatment response to systemic therapy. For reference, the staging schema for gastric and non-gastric GISTs is shown in table 2 of American Joint Committee on Cancer Staging Manual 8th Edition, 2017.[44]

Management of clinically relevant, localized GIST consists of resection with or without adjuvant targeted therapy with the tyrosine kinase inhibitor (TKI) imatinib mesylate.[3,42] Complete surgical excision without lymph node dissection should be performed following the principles of oncologic surgery to achieve a margin microscopically free of tumor cells (R0 resection). For gastric lesions, this commonly involves a segmental or wedge resection without tumor rupture, as rupture greatly increases the risk of peritoneal recurrence. For small intestinal or colonic GISTs, segmental resection of the involved segment of bowel without lymphadenectomy should suffice. If the scope of surgery would lead to major functional sequalae or is otherwise not feasible, neoadjuvant targeted therapy with imatinib may be pursued in tumors with sensitive mutations (see Section 3). In particular, GISTs arising in the esophagus, duodenum, or rectum (which might require an esophagectomy, pancreaticoduodenectomy, or abdominoperineal resection) may benefit from a course of neoadjuvant imatinib to enable a more limited esophageal, duodenal, or transanal resection, respectively.

PROGNOSTIC FACTORS AND RISK OF RECURRENCE

Several key prognostic factors are used in models for recurrence that identify tumors at high risk of relapse and guide the decision to pursue adjuvant therapy with imatinib. Tumor size, mitotic rate, and tumor site are the key prognostic factors as confirmed in multiple models, and tumor rupture is frequently thought to be an independent prognostic factor as well (**Table 2**).[45–48]

The most likely sites of recurrence or distant metastasis are the peritoneum and liver. Metastases to bone are rare and local recurrences are not the usual pattern of recurrence for adult-type GISTs. Recurrence or progression typically occurs within one to 3 years after resection or completion of adjuvant therapy.[3] In general, guidelines for surveillance are based on the risk of recurrence.[3,42] For very low- and low-risk tumors not requiring adjuvant therapy, patients may be followed with an abdominal CT initially every 3 to 6 months for 2 years, then every 6 to 12 months for the next 3 years and then annually. For intermediate- or high-risk tumors, patients may be followed with abdominal CT every 3 months for 2 years during adjuvant therapy, then every 6 months for an additional 3 years, and then annually.

ADJUVANT THERAPY

Before the advent of adjuvant therapy, recurrence and survival after complete resection were approximately 40% and 54% at 5 years, respectively.[49] The development of targeted therapy with the TKI imatinib for use in advanced GIST led to the investigation of imatinib in the adjuvant setting for patients with localized GIST at risk of recurrence.

Several prospective trials phase 2 and phase 3 trials have evaluated the role of imatinib for 1, 2, 3, or 5 years following complete resection.[3,45,50,51] All trials have shown that adjuvant therapy improved recurrence-free survival (RFS) rates. The phase 3 trial evaluating 3 years versus 1 year of adjuvant imatinib confirmed that a longer duration

Table 2 Modified National Institutes of Health Risk Stratification criteria for GIST			
Risk category	Tumor size (cm)	Mitotic index (per 50 HPFs)	Primary tumor site
Very low risk	< 2.0	≤ 5	Any
Low risk	2.1–5.0	≤ 5	Any
Intermediate risk	2.1–5.0	> 5	Gastric
	< 5.0	6–10	Any
	5.1–10.0	≤ 5	Gastric
High risk	Any	Any	Tumor rupture
	> 10 cm	Any	Any
	Any	> 10	Any
	> 5.0	> 5	Any
	2.1–5.0	> 5	Nongastric

Modified NIH risk stratification criteria for GIST with rupture included.
Abbreviation: GIST, gastrointestinal stromal tumor; HPF, high power fields; NIH, National Institutes of Health.
Reproduced from: Joensuu H. Risk stratification of patients diagnosed with gastrointestinal stromal tumor. Hum Pathol 2008; 39:1411. Table used with permission of Elsevier Inc. All rights reserved.

of therapy also improved overall survival (OS). Importantly, these studies have demonstrated that adjuvant imatinib therapy is most beneficial in patients with prognostic factors predictive of a high recurrence risk and with imatinib-sensitive mutations, such as *KIT* exon 11 deletion.[3,50,51] Tumors with *KIT* exon 9 or *PDGRA* D842 V mutations or GISTs that are *KIT/PDGFRA* wild-type, *NF1*-related, or SDH-deficient do not appear to benefit from imatinib.[3]

The phase 2 single-arm 5-year study confirmed that disease control was maintained in patients with sensitive mutations although they remained on imatinib.[51] Once imatinib was discontinued, the risk of recurrence was highest in the following 2 years.

Most recent clinical trials with adjuvant imatinib have demonstrated RFS of 65.6% to 90% and OS of 92% to 95% at 5 years.[50,51] The current standard of care is to offer patients with high risk (and in some countries, including the US, moderate risk) at least 3 years of adjuvant imatinib (based on the longest duration phase 3 trial). Ongoing phase 3 trials are looking at a longer duration therapy. Notably, all the adjuvant trials have demonstrated progressively higher elective drug discontinuation rates by patients with progressively longer durations of therapy, stressing the importance of close follow-up during therapy.[3,45,50,51]

NEOADJUVANT THERAPY

Neoadjuvant therapy before surgery should be considered in patients in whom tumor size reduction would decrease the morbidity of resection, increase organ preservation, and facilitate complete oncologic resection (R0 resection) for a tumor with an amenable mutational profile.[42,52,53] For example, neoadjuvant therapy for large gastric GISTs could result in an interval size reduction to facilitate segmental resection instead of gastrectomy and potentially enable resection through a minimally invasive (laparascopic or robotic) approach. Consideration for neoadjuvant therapy would include patients with either locally advanced or marginal/borderline resectable tumors. Imatinib-sensitive mutations have been highlighted in the previous sections. Avapritinib could hypothetically be used for *PDGFRA* exon 18D842 V mutations although it has not been formally evaluated in a *neoadjuvant* trial for primary, resectable GIST.[42] The use of neoadjuvant therapy before complete pathologic evaluation at the time of surgery precludes the ability to obtain a reliable mitotic count, a prognostic factor for recurrence risk stratification. Pretreatment biopsy may help determine the tumor's mutational profile and guide the neoadjuvant regimen but does not necessarily accurately predict mitotic count. If prognostic recurrence risk cannot be predicted, then patients treated with neadjuvant imatinib typically are committed to a course of 3 years of imatinib (neoadjuvant plus adjuvant).

Two trials provide guidance about the use of neoadjuvant therapy in locally advanced GISTs. The RTOG 0132/ACRIN 6665 trial, a single-phase II United States Intergroup trial, treated resectable primary GISTs greater than or equal to 5 cm or a resectable recurrence with neoadjuvant imatinib for 8 to 12 weeks.[54] 7% of cases had an objective response on neoadjuvant therapy, whereas 83% had stable disease. A phase II Asian trial treated gastric GISTs greater than or equal to 10 cm with neoadjuvant imatinib for 6 to 9 months.[55] Maximal tumor size reduction was noted at 3 months in 20% of tumors, 6 months in 63% of tumors, and 9 months in 15% of tumors. R0 resection was achieved in 91% of cases with preservation of greater than half of the stomach in 88% of cases. Two-year OS and progression-free survival were 98% and 89%, respectively. Given the results of these trials, it is recommended that neoadjuvant therapy should be given for at least 6 months and potentially up to 12 months or as long as the tumor exhibits continued radiographic response.[3]

Given the protracted course of neoadjuvant treatment required, a serial response assessment throughout this time interval is necessary. A baseline PET or CT should be obtained before treatment initiation, if not done previously as part of initial tumor staging, and then throughout treatment (usually just CT alone; routine PET is not necessary but may be indicated in select patients).[3,42] With treatment, large tumors may initially increase in size early during the course, theorized to be due to intratumoral hemorrhage or myxoid degeneration. Subsequently, the lesion may decrease in density on CT or FDG uptake on PET and then eventually decrease in size before stabilization. In late responders, the tumor will show stability for the initial 6 months, whereas in nonresponders, the tumor will demonstrate an absence of response. Alternate therapy should be considered for nonresponders.

METASTATIC GASTROINTESTINAL STROMAL TUMORS

For metastatic GIST, receptor TKIs are the standard therapy.[3,42] More specifically, imatinib 400 mg daily is the first-line treatment for sensitive mutations. Certain mutations require alternative dosing, such as the *KIT* exon 9 mutation (imatinib 800 mg is recommended) or an alternate agent such as for a *PDGFRA* D842 V mutation (avapritinib is recommended). Therapy should be administered as long as there is a treatment response or stable disease. If no response, generalized progression, or complete therapeutic intolerance occurs on first-line therapy, the following sequence should be applied in succession after each escalation in therapy is deemed unsuccessful: increase imatinib dose, transition to sunitinib as second-line therapy, transition to regorafenib as third-line therapy, and transition to ripretinib as fourth-line therapy. Additional therapeutics, such as sorafenib, dasatinib, nilotinib, pazopanib, and everolimus in combination with a TKI, exist for progression on the above lines of therapy and should be selected on an individualized case basis.[42] Alternatively, responses are occasionally seen following rechallenge of a previously tolerated TKI.[3]

Therapy should be continued if there is a treatment response as it provides symptom palliation and, with cessation of therapy, a flare response with disease progression occurs.[56]

Once systemic therapy is initiated, surveillance abdominal imaging with CT or MRI should be performed every 8 to 12 weeks to assess for progression.[3,42] Progression includes a new lesion, an increase in tumor size, or a "nodule within a mass" in which a portion of the tumor becomes hyperdense. False progression may be seen with therapy noncompliance, drug interactions, or with indeterminate response patterns. Lesion density evaluation or PET/CT may be used to clarify ambiguity.

Although prospective trials examining the role of surgery in advanced disease failed to accrue and thus efficacy cannot be determined, surgical metastatectomy during systemic therapy may be considered in select clinical scenarios. Surgery on residual disease may be indicated after initiation of imatinib (at least 6–12 months) with either a disease response, stable disease, or a progressing lesion with limited nonmultifocal progression.[3] Retrospective studies have shown that surgery in nonmultifocal progression results in a similar progression-free survival as that of the second-line therapy.[57] The morbidity of resection may be predicted by preoperative surgical complexity scores and is typically worse after an incomplete resection.[42,58] Common complications include superficial or deep tissue infection, anastomotic leak, ileus or obstruction, bleeding, venous thromboembolism, and pneumonia.

SUMMARY

The management of GISTs depends on the stage of the tumor—small, clinically relevant localized, locally advanced, or metastatic. For small GISTs of the intestine and gastric GISTs with high-risk features, surgery is recommended. Clinically relevant and localized GISTs warrant oncologic resection followed by adjuvant targeted therapy for lesions with intermediate to high recurrence risk with mutation-sensitive chemotherapeutic agents administered for at least 3 years. For locally advanced GISTs, neoadjuvant therapy should be considered for at least 6 months before oncologic resection for tumors in which a size reduction would decrease the morbidity of resection, increase organ preservation, or facilitate complete oncologic resection. For metastatic GISTs, targeted therapy is the standard of care; surgery may be an appropriate consideration for patients with metastatic GIST on systemic therapy with a disease response, stable disease, or limited nonmultifocal progression.

CLINICS CARE POINTS

- The diagnostic modality of choice for GISTs is an EUS with fine-needle aspiration or biopsy, which demonstrates characteristic features of an elastic, firm, well-demarcated, hypoechoic lesion. Oral and intravenous contrast-enhanced abdominal and pelvic CT, with characteristic findings of a solid enhancing lesion with smooth contours, is the cross-sectional technique of choice for primary tumor characterization.

- The goals of resection are a macroscopically complete resection with negative microscopic margins (R0 resection) without lymph node dissection and prevention of tumor rupture to avoid tumor seeding and intraperitoneal contamination

- Tumor size, mitotic rate, tumor site, and tumor rupture are key prognostic factors that determine tumor recurrence with the most likely sites of recurrence or distant metastasis being the peritoneum and liver.

- Surveillance necessitates serial abdominal CT at varying intervals depending on the risk of recurrence and time from resection.
- Adjuvant therapy with TKI imatinib in tumor-sensitive mutations in high recurrence risk tumors improves OS when administered for at least 3 years after resection. Tumors with *KIT* exon 9 or *PDGFRA* D842 V mutations or GISTs that are *KIT/PDGFRA* wild type, NF1-related, or SDH-deficient do not appear to benefit from imatinib.
- In appropriate cases, neoadjuvant therapy should be given for at least 6 months and potentially up to 12 months or as long as the tumor exhibits continued radiographic response with serial response assessment.
- For metastatic GIST, imatinib 400 mg daily is the first-line treatment for sensitive mutations. If no response, generalized progression, or complete therapeutic intolerance occurs on first-line therapy, increase imatinib dose, transition to sunitinib as second-line therapy, transition to regorafenib as third-line therapy, and transition to ripretinib as fourth-line therapy. Surgery with metastatectomy may be considered in select clinical scenarios.

DISCLOSURE

The authors have nothing to disclose.

REFERENCES

1. Hong NJL, Raut CP. Gastrointestinal stromal tumors. In: Zinner MJ, Ashley SW, Hines OJ, editors. Maingot's abdominal operations. 13rd edition. New York, (NY): McGraw-Hill Education; 2019.
2. Søreide K, Sandvik OM, Søreide JA, et al. Global epidemiology of gastrointestinal stromal tumours (GIST): a systematic review of population-based cohort studies. Cancer Epidemiol 2016;40:39–46.
3. Casali PG, Abecassis N, Bauer S, et al. Gastrointestinal stromal tumours: ESMO–EURACAN Clinical Practice Guidelines for diagnosis, treatment and follow-up. Ann Oncol 2018;29:iv68–78.
4. Tran T, Davila JA, El-Serag HB. The epidemiology of malignant gastrointestinal stromal tumors: an analysis of 1,458 cases from 1992 to 2000. Am J Gastroenterol 2005;100(1):162–8.
5. Hirota S, Isozaki K, Moriyama Y, et al. Gain-of-function mutations of c-kit in human gastrointestinal stromal tumors. Science 1998;279(5350):577–80.
6. Schaefer IM, Wang Y, Liang CW, et al. MAX inactivation is an early event in GIST development that regulates p16 and cell proliferation. Nat Commun 2017; 8(1):1–6.
7. Carney JA. June). Gastric stromal sarcoma, pulmonary chondroma, and extra-adrenal paraganglioma (Carney Triad): natural history, adrenocortical component, and possible familial occurrence. Mayo Clinic Proc 1999;74(No. 6): 543–52. Elsevier.
8. Stratakis CA, Carney JA. The triad of paragangliomas, gastric stromal tumours and pulmonary chondromas (Carney triad), and the dyad of paragangliomas and gastric stromal sarcomas (Carney–Stratakis syndrome): molecular genetics and clinical implications. J Intern Med 2009;266(1):43–52.
9. Miettinen M, Fetsch JF, Sobin LH, et al. Gastrointestinal stromal tumors in patients with neurofibromatosis 1: a clinicopathologic and molecular genetic study of 45 cases. Am J Surg Pathol 2006;30(1):90–6.

10. Andersson J, Sihto H, Meis-Kindblom JM, et al. NF1-associated gastrointestinal stromal tumors have unique clinical, phenotypic, and genotypic characteristics. Am J Surg Pathol 2005;29(9):1170-6.

11. Maeyama H, Hidaka E, Ota H, et al. Familial gastrointestinal stromal tumor with hyperpigmentation: association with a germline mutation of the c-kit gene. Gastroenterology 2001;120(1):210-5.

12. Kawanowa K, Sakuma Y, Sakurai S, et al. High incidence of micro- scopic gastro-intestinal stromal tumors in the stomach. Hum Pathol 2006;37:1527-35.

13. Abraham SC, Krasinskas AM, Hofstetter WL, et al. Seedling" mes- enchymal tumors (gastrointestinal stromal tumors and leiomyomas) are common incidental tumors of the esophagogastric junction. Am J Surg Pathol 2007;31:1629-35.

14. Rossi S, Gasparotto D, Toffolatti L, et al. Molecular and clinico- pathologic characterization of gastrointestinal stromal tumors (GISTs) of small size. Am J Surg Pathol 2010;34:1480-91.

15. Nishida T, Goto O, Raut CP, et al. Diagnostic and treatment strategy for small gastrointestinal stromal tumors. Cancer 2016;122(20):3110-8.

16. Sakamoto H, Kitano M, Matsui S, et al. Estimation of malignant potential of GI stromal tumors by contrast-enhanced harmonic EUS (with videos). Gastrointest Endosc 2011;73:227-37.

17. Tsuji Y, Kusano C, Gotoda T, et al. Diagnostic potential of endo- scopic ultrasonography-elastography for gastric submucosal tumors: a pilot study. Dig Endosc 2016;28:173-8.

18. Nishida T, Hirota S, Yanagisawa A, et al. Clinical practice guidelines for gastrointestinal stromal tumor (GIST) in Japan: English version. Int J Clin Oncol 2008;13: 416-30.

19. Rosch T, Kapfer B, Will U, et al. Accuracy of endoscopic ultraso- nography in upper gastrointestinal submucosal lesions: a prospective multicenter study. Scand J Gastroenterol 2002;7:856-62.

20. Ponsaing LG, Kiss K, Loft A, et al. Diagnostic procedures for sub- mucosal tumors in the gastrointestinal tract. World J Gastroenterol 2007;13:3301-10.

21. Demetri GD, von Mehren M, Antonescu CR, et al. NCCN Task Force report: update on the management of patients with gastroin- testinal stromal tumors. J Natl Compr Canc Netw 2010;8(suppl 2):S1-41.

22. Lee M, Min BH, Lee H, et al. Feasibility and diagnostic yield of endoscopic ultrasonography-guided fine needle biopsy with a new core biopsy needle device in patients with gastric subepithelial tumors. Medicine (Baltimore) 2015;94(40): e1622.

23. Trindade AJ, Benias PC, Alshelleh M, et al. Fine-needle biopsy is superior to fine-needle aspiration of suspected gastrointestinal stromal tumors: a large multi-center study. Endosc Int Open 2019;7(07):E931-6.

24. Yamabe A, Irisawa A, Bhutani MS, et al. Usefulness of endoscopic ultrasound-guided fine-needle aspiration with a forward-viewing and curved linear-array echoendoscope for small gastrointestinal subepi- thelial lesions [serial online]. Endosc Int Open 2015;3:E161-4.

25. Agaimy A, Wunsch PH, Hofstaedter F, et al. Minute gastric scleros- ing stromal tumors (GIST tumorlets) are common in adults and fre- quently show c-KIT mutations. Am J Surg Pathol 2007;31:113-20.

26. Agaimy A, Wunsch PH, Dirnhofer S, et al. Microscopic gastrointes- tinal stromal tumors in esophageal and intestinal surgical resection specimens: a clinicopath-ologic, immunohistochemical, and molecular study of 19 lesions. Am J Surg Pathol 2008;32:867-73.

27. Antonescu CR, Viale A, Sarran L, et al. Gene expression in gastroin- testinal stro-mal tumors is distinguished by KIT genotype and ana- tomic site. Clin Cancer Res 2004;10:3282–90.
28. Nishida T, Kawai N, Yamaguchi S, et al. Submucosal tumors: com- prehensive guide for the diagnosis and therapy of gastrointestinal submucosal tumors. Dig Endosc 2013;25:479–89.
29. Sawaki A, Mizuno N, Takahashi K, et al. Long-term follow up of patients with small gastrointestinal stromal tumors in the stomach using endoscopic ultrasonography-guided fine-needle aspiration biop- sy. Dig Endosc 2006; 18:40–4.
30. Sekine M, Imaoka H, Mizuno N, et al. Clinical course of gastroin- testinal stromal tumor diagnosed by endoscopic ultrasound-guided fine-needle aspiration. Dig Endosc 2015;27:44–52.
31. Novitsky YW, Kercher KW, Sing RF, et al. Long-term outcomes of laparoscopic resection of gastric gastrointestinal stromal tumors. Ann Surg 2006;243:738–45.
32. Nishimura J, Nakajima K, Omori T, et al. Surgical strategy for gas- tric gastroin-testinal stromal tumors: laparoscopic vs open resection. Surg Endosc 2007;21: 875–8.
33. Bischof DA, Kim Y, Dodson R, et al. Open versus minimally inva- sive resection of gastric GIST: a multi-institutional analysis of short- and long-term outcomes. Ann Surg Oncol 2014;21:2941–8.
34. Chen K, Zhou YC, Mou YP, et al. Systematic review and meta- analysis of safety and efficacy of laparoscopic resection for gastrointes- tinal stromal tumors of the stomach. Surg Endosc 2015;29:355–67.
35. Hiki N, Yamamoto Y, Fukunaga T, et al. Laparoscopic and endo- scopic cooper-ative surgery for gastrointestinal stromal tumor dissec- tion. Surg Endosc 2008; 22:1729–35.
36. Abe N, Takeuchi H, Yanagida O, et al. Endoscopic full-thickness re- section with laparoscopic assistance as hybrid NOTES for gastric submucosal tumor. Surg Endosc 2009;23:1908–13.
37. Hoteya S, Haruta S, Shinohara H, et al. Feasibility and safety of lap- aroscopic and endoscopic cooperative surgery for gastric submucosal tumors, including esophagogastric junction tumors. Dig Endosc 2014;26:538–44.
38. Nilsson B, Bumming P, Meis-Kindblom JM, et al. Gastrointestinal stro- mal tumors: the incidence, prevalence, clinical course, and prognostica- tion in the preimati-nib mesylate era–a population-based study in western Sweden. Cancer 2005; 103:821–9.
39. American Cancer Society. Key statistics for gastrointestinal stromal tumors amer-ican cancer society. 2019 [Available at: https://www.cancer.org/cancer/ gastrointestinal-stromal-tumor/about/key-statistics.html.
40. Caterino S, Lorenzon L, Petrucciani N, et al. Gastrointestinal stromal tumors: cor-relation between symptoms at presentation, tumor location and prognostic fac-tors in 47 consecutive patients. World J Surg Oncol 2011;9:13.
41. Graadt van Roggen JF, van Velthuysen ML, Hogendoorn PC. The histopatholog-ical differential diagnosis of gastrointestinal stromal tumours. J Clin Pathol 2001; 54(2):96–102.
42. National Comprehensive Cancer Network. Gastrointestinal stromal tumors (GIST) version 1.2021. Plymouth Meeting (PA): NCCN.org; 2020.
43. Watson RR, Binmoeller KF, Hamerski CM, et al. Yield and performance character-istics of endoscopic ultrasound-guided fine needle aspiration for diagnosing up-per GI tract stromal tumors. Dig Dis Sci 2011;56(6):1757–62.

44. Amin MB, Greene FL, Edge SB, et al. The eighth edition AJCC cancer staging manual: continuing to build a bridge from a population-based to a more "personalized" approach to cancer staging. CA Cancer J Clin 2017;67(2):93–9.
45. Dematteo RP, Gold JS, Saran L, et al. Tumor mitotic rate, size, and location independently predict recurrence after resection of primary gastrointestinal stromal tumor (GIST). Cancer 2008;112(3):608–15.
46. Huang HY, Li CF, Huang WW, et al. A modification of NIH consensus criteria to better distinguish the highly lethal subset of primary localized gastrointestinal stromal tumors: a subdivision of the original high-risk group on the basis of outcome. Surgery 2007;141(6):748–56.
47. Gold JS, Gönen M, Gutiérrez A, et al. Development and validation of a prognostic nomogram for recurrence-free survival after complete surgical resection of localised primary gastrointestinal stromal tumour: a retrospective analysis. Lancet Oncol 2009;10(11):1045–52.
48. Rossi S, Miceli R, Messerini L, et al. Natural history of imatinib-naive GISTs: a retrospective analysis of 929 cases with long-term follow-up and development of a survival nomogram based on mitotic index and size as continuous variables. Am J Surg Pathol 2011;35(11):1646–56.
49. DeMatteo RP, Lewis JJ, Leung D, et al. Two hundred gastrointestinal stromal tumors: recurrence patterns and prognostic factors for survival. Ann Surg 2000; 231(1):51.
50. Joensuu H, Eriksson M, Sundby Hall K, et al. One vs three years of adjuvant imatinib for operable gastrointestinal stromal tumor: a randomized trial. JAMA 2012; 307(12):1265–72.
51. Raut CP, Espat NJ, Maki RG, et al. Efficacy and tolerability of 5-year adjuvant imatinib treatment for patients with resected intermediate- or high-risk primary gastrointestinal stromal tumor: the PERSIST-5 clinical trial. JAMA Oncol 2018; 4(12):e184060.
52. von Mehren M, Watson JC. Perioperative tyrosine kinase inhibitors for GIST: standard… or an idea that needs further investigation? Oncology (Williston Park) 2009;23(1):65.
53. Gronchi A, Raut CP. The combination of surgery and imatinib in GIST: a reality for localized tumors at high risk, an open issue for metastatic ones. Ann Surg Oncol 2012;19(4):1051–5.
54. Eisenberg BL, Harris J, Blanke CD, et al. Phase II trial of neoadjuvant/adjuvant imatinib mesylate (IM) for advanced primary and metastatic/recurrent operable gastrointestinal stromal tumor (GIST): early results of RTOG 0132/ACRIN 6665. J Surg Oncol 2009;99(1):42–7.
55. Kurokawa Y, Yang HK, Cho H, et al. Phase II study of neoadjuvant imatinib in large gastrointestinal stromal tumours of the stomach. Br J Cancer 2017; 117(1):25–32.
56. Patrikidou A, Le Cesne A. Key messages from the BFR14 trial of the French Sarcoma Group. Future Oncol 2017;13(3):273–84.
57. Fairweather M, Balachandran VP, Li GZ, et al. Cytoreductive Surgery for Metastatic Gastrointestinal Stromal Tumors Treated with Tyrosine Kinase Inhibitors: A Two Institutional Analysis. Ann Surg 2018;268(2):296.
58. Fairweather M, Cavnar MJ, Li GZ, et al. Prediction of morbidity following cytoreductive surgery for metastatic gastrointestinal stromal tumour in patients on tyrosine kinase inhibitor therapy. J Br Surg 2018;105(6):743–50.

Lipoma and Its Doppelganger
The Atypical Lipomatous Tumor/Well-Differentiated Liposarcoma

Elliott J. Yee, MD[a],*, Camille L. Stewart, MD[a],
Michael R. Clay, MD[b], Martin M. McCarter, MD[a]

KEYWORDS

- Lipoma • Well-differentiated liposarcoma • Diagnosis • Management • Review

KEY POINTS

- Differentiation between a benign lipoma and an atypical lipomatous tumor/well-differentiated liposarcoma presents a diagnostic challenge.
- Magnetic resonance imaging and computed tomography are the gold standard imaging modalities for extremity and peritoneal lipomas/liposarcomas, respectively.
- First-line therapy for benign lipomas and low-grade liposarcomas is surgical excision.
- Retroperitoneal low-grade liposarcomas have a higher propensity for local recurrence, histologic dedifferentiation, and mortality compared with extremity counterparts.

INTRODUCTION

Soft tissue masses (STMs) are among the most common pathologic conditions encountered by the general surgeon. Benign lipomatous tumors, better known as lipomas, account for the vast majority of STMs. However, atypical lipomatous tumors (ALT)/well-differentiated liposarcomas (WDLPS), low grade but locally aggressive soft tissue sarcomas (STSs) with a propensity for recurrence and ability to dedifferentiate, make up nearly 10% of all STMs.[1,2] Differentiating a benign lipoma from an ALT/WDLPS often presents a diagnostic dilemma with important therapeutic and prognostic implications. Although a detailed history of present illness and thorough physical examination of, for example, a slow-growing subcutaneous lump or a distended abdomen with associated unexplained weight gain, can provide critical information, they are often insufficient to make a definitive diagnosis. Moreover, even with the

[a] Department of Surgery, University of Colorado, 12605 East 16th Avenue, Aurora, CO 80045, USA; [b] Department of Pathology, Univeristy of Colorado, 12605 East 16th Avenue, Aurora, CO 80045, USA
* Corresponding author.
E-mail address: elliott.yee@cuanschutz.edu

Surg Clin N Am 102 (2022) 637–656
https://doi.org/10.1016/j.suc.2022.04.006
0039-6109/22/© 2022 Elsevier Inc. All rights reserved.
surgical.theclinics.com

Abbreviations	
WDLPS	Well-differentiated liposarcoma
STM	Soft tissue mass
ALT	A typical lipomatous lesion

help of advanced imaging modalities, separation of benign from malignant is not guaranteed. For these reasons, we refer to ALT/WDLPS as a doppelganger, or look-a-like, to the lipoma—to the trained and untrained eye alike, the liposarcoma is a sinister lesion that can masquerade as its less aggressive counterpart, confusing all who examine it. Nevertheless, with a dedicated investigation and well-rounded knowledge of these two seemingly mirror pathologic conditions, accurate diagnosis of these two lesions can be achieved and treated accordingly.

This article will review and juxtapose the epidemiology, diagnosis, management, natural history, and surveillance strategies of benign lipomas and ALT/WDLPS. In addition, we aim to highlight aspects of each topic relevant to the general surgical community at large with an emphasis for those that practice outside of the subspecialty setting.

Epidemiology/Nomenclature

Lipomas are ubiquitous. They are the most common STM occurring in 1% to 2% of the population. The reported incidence of lipomas is 2 per 1000 people per year; however, the true incidence is likely much higher secondary to underreporting.[3,4] These well-defined adipocytic tumors can arise in any age group but generally appear in the fourth to sixth decade of life without apparent gender predilection.[3,5] Compared with all liposarcomas, lipomas are 100 times more common.[4] Proposed risk factors for lipomas include genetic predisposition and local trauma (**Table 1**).[6,7]

As of the 2020 fifth edition of the World Health Organization Classification of Soft Tissue and Bone Tumors, WDLPS is classified as 1 of 4 official variants of liposarcoma (others being dedifferentiated, myxoid/round cell, and pleomorphic) and 1 of more than 50 histologic subtypes of STS.[8] This entity has been further divided into ALT and WDLPS based on tumor location, surgical resectability, and propensity for dedifferentiation despite identical histologic and molecular features.[9] ALT refers to tumors occurring on the extremities, truncal region, and abdominal wall, whereas the designation of WDLPS is reserved for those arising in deep-seated locations such as the retroperitoneum, mediastinum, and paratesticular region. The proximity of WDLPS to surrounding structures compromises resectability and thus results in twice the local recurrence rate, 10 times the risk of histologic dedifferentiation, and greater disease-specific mortality as compared with ALT.[2,10,11] ALT/WDLPS represent about half of all liposarcomas.[2] Because the retroperitoneum is composed of a relative abundance of

Table 1
Epidemiologic differences between lipoma and atypical lipomatous tumor/well-differentiated liposarcomas[6,15]

	Lipoma	ALT/WDLPS
Population incidence	2 per 1000 per year	0.35 per 100,000 per year
Age at diagnosis	Any; 30–50 year old	50–60 year old
Sex	M = F	M > F
Risk factors for development	Genetic, trauma	Unknown

fatty tissue, liposarcomas occurring in this compartment are a hallmark of the disease, accounting for about 12% of all STS and a third of all tumors arising from the retroperitoneum.[12,13] A total of 50% of retroperitoneal liposarcomas are of the well-differentiated subtype.[12,14] Compared with lipomas, ALT/WDLPS have a slight male predominance (1.5:1), affect Caucasians 10 times more than African-Americans and are typically diagnosed during the sixth–seventh decade of life.[15,16] Although prior radiation and occupational exposures (eg, vinyl chloride in plastics manufacturing) predispose to some forms of soft tissue/vascular sarcomas, clear causative/risk factors have not been correlated with the development of ALT/WDLPS.[17]

Diagnosis

History of present illness and physical examination
Although accurate distinction of a benign lipoma from the more aggressive ALT/WDLPS cannot solely rely on a thorough history and physical assessment alone, it must begin with one. Pertinent questions to ask patients presenting with an STM arising from the extremity/trunk or peritoneum/retroperitoneum should follow conventional queries of onset, duration, symptomatology, associated factors, and past medical and familial histories. A history of recurring subcutaneous lesions may indicate a potentially aggressive/malignant process rather than a benign lesion. A focused physical examination of a focal peripheral lesion or the abdomen can glean much information about the patient's pathologic condition. Examples of questions to guide physical assessment focus on characteristics of the mass and its surroundings—how large or deep is the mass, can it be palpated free of its surrounding structures, what are the surrounding structures, is the abdomen distended, is there a palpable abdominal mass?

Lipomas can occur anywhere on the body but are most commonly found at the proximal extremities and abdominal wall/truncal region.[2,4] Most lipomas are located superficially in the subcutaneous tissue but 1% to 2% of cases occur as deep, subfascial tumors in the chest wall or as inter/intramuscular extremity lipomas.[18,19] About 85% of superficial lipomas are less than 5 cm in diameter, whereas ALTs average 15 cm on initial presentation.[1,15] Both peripherally located lipomas and ALT are generally slow-growing, painless, well-circumscribed masses, described as "dough-like" in consistency, which typically present to the clinician after months to years of steady enlargement.[20] Compression of nearby structures, namely nerves and vessels, can present as a pressure-like sensation but rarely as overt pain. Multiple lipomas are found in 5% to 15% of people affected by lipomas. These can occur in a sporadic fashion such as in Madelung disease (benign symmetric lipomatosis[21]), and adiposa dolorosa (a rare condition characterized by the growth of multiple, painful lipomas[22]) or secondary to inherited genetic abnormalities such as Cowden syndrome, Bannayan-Zonana syndrome, Frohlich syndrome, and neurofibromatosis type 1.[3,4] **Table 2** outlines clinical characteristics, with varying degrees of sensitivity and/or specificity, in differentiating lipoma and ALT/WDLPS, which should be used as guides rather than rules when faced with a soft tissue lesion arising from the extremity location.

In contrast, intra-abdominal lipomas and retroperitoneal WDLPS occur less frequently than their extremity/trunk counterparts.[23] Intra-abdominal lipomas can arise from the soft tissue of the retroperitoneum, directly from visceral organs, and/or from the mesentery (**Fig. 1**). Retroperitoneal lipomas are rare entities with less than 50 case reports published since the 1970s; however, similar to lipomas in general, the incidence is likely severely underreported.[24] Of note, spermatic cord lipomas, fat collections within a hernia sac commonly encountered during indirect hernia

Table 2
Examination and radiologic differences among lipoma, atypical lipomatous tumor, and well-differentiated liposarcomas[4]

	Lipoma	ALT	WDLPS
Anatomic location	Any	LE > UE > trunk > head and neck	Retroperitoneum, mediastinum, paratesticular
Size at diagnosis (avg, cm)	<5 (1% are >10)	14	18
Relationship to surrounding structures	Well-circumscribed, subcutaneous, 1% are deep	Compression of nearby structures	"Pushing" vs invading viscera
Radiologic findings			
Ultrasound	Discrete hyperechoic mass; homogenous	Complex, hyperechoic mass; moderate internal heterogeneity, multilobulated	
MRI	Isointense to subcutaneous fat, no contrast enhancement; thin septa (<2 mm)	Septal enhancement; thick septa (>2 mm); nodular/patchy nonadipose components	
CT	Discrete, homogenous mass; simple fat attenuation, lack septa	Simple fat attenuating mass, thick/nodular enhancing septa	Displaced organs ± invasion; predominantly simple fat attenuation; thin to thick septa

Abbreviations: LE, lower extremity; UE, upper extremity.

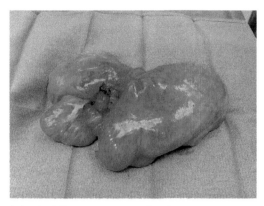

Fig. 1. Large intra-abdominal lipoma, gross specimen.

repairs, are not true "lipomas" because they are not tumors of fat cells but rather simple preperitoneal fat tracking in the inguinal canal.[25] Retroperitoneal liposarcomas make up 12% to 15% of STS, half of which are well-differentiated or dedifferentiated liposarcoma subtypes.[12] Clinical presentation of benign and locally aggressive intra-abdominal adipocytic lesions are characterized by a feeling of intra-abdominal fullness, nonspecific abdominal pain, unintended weight gain, sciatica, and rarely signs and symptoms of bowel obstruction—most of these are consequences of mass effect and compression of nearby structures. A large population-based analysis found that the average size of retroperitoneal WDLPS was 18 cm.[16] This is a testament to the clinically silent nature of these tumors, which can be present without significant symptoms for long periods of time because these are often "pushing" tumors rather than tumors that invade into adjacent structures. Similarly, retroperitoneal lipomas as large as 55 cm have been reported.[26] Although ALTs are conventionally thought to be faster growing than lipomas, actual growth rates of primary abdominal lipomas and WDLPS are unknown.

Imaging

Imaging is often valuable for the presurgical assessment of both lipomas and ALT/WDLPS and can frequently delineate lipoma from ALT/WDLPS (see **Table 2**). Thus, bedside and advanced cross-sectional imaging modalities are the next component in the workup of an undifferentiated soft tissue lesion. Obtaining imaging studies should be considered in deep-seated lesions and those more than 5 cm in size. Ultrasonography (US) is often an inexpensive, low-risk study that conveys gross characteristics of a subcutaneous lesion such as estimation of size, location relative to fascia, echogenicity and heterogeneity of tissue, and regularity of borders. Unfortunately, sensitivity and specificity of US in differentiating lipoma from ALT/WDLPS is poor because both lipomas and ALT/WDLPS can demonstrate heterogeneity, hyperechogenicity suggestive of fat and/or septa, varying depths relative to underlying fascia, and multilobulation.[27]

Multiphase magnetic resonance imaging (MRI) with or without contrast is the gold standard specifically for the evaluation of extremity STM.[28] The ability of MRI to delineate bone, soft tissue, and vascular structures makes it well-suited to characterize tumor proximity to clinically relevant structures. Further, radiologic comparison studies using MRI have demonstrated consistent differences between lipomas and ALT/WDLPS. ALT/WDLPS are often greater than 10 cm in maximum diameter, have thicker, more contrast-enhancing septa on T2-weighted images, and are more likely

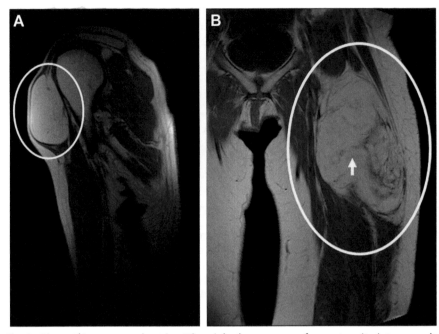

Fig. 2. Magnetic resonance imaging T2-weighed sequences of an extremity intramuscular lipoma (*A*) and ALT (*B*). Yellow circles denote location of the tumor. Note for the atypical lipomatous tumor the larger size, thicker and more contrast-enhancing septa (*arrow*), and lower adipose composition of the tumor.

to have 75% or less of tumor volume made of adipose tissue (**Fig. 2**).[27,29–31] With these criteria, MRI reaches 100% and 83% sensitivity and specificity, respectively, in differentiating benign lipomas from ALT/WDLPS.[32] Gadolinium administration can be particularly useful as a screening examination for WDLPS as contrast enhancement has a sensitivity of 100% but specificity and positive predictive value of only 71% and 53%, respectively.[33]

Computed tomography (CT) with intravenous contrast is the modality of choice for evaluation of intra-abdominal/retroperitoneal lesions as it can best characterize the relationship between the tumor and the adjacent displaced visceral organs. Fatty tumors within the retroperitoneum clearly not arising from solid or hollow abdominal structures and associated with displaced organs are suggestive of liposarcoma because most WDLPS are considered "pushing" as opposed to invasive tumors (**Fig. 3**).[34] Both intra-abdominal lipomas and WDLPS often demonstrate simple fat attenuation (Hounsfield units −10 to −100). CT imaging of the chest and pelvis can appropriately stage a tumor in addition to providing baseline studies for surveillance of metastatic disease. Currently, there is no role for PET/CT in the diagnosis, characterization, or differentiation between lipomas and more aggressive soft tissue lesions.[35,36]

Biopsy
A biopsy before definitive management is often essential in differentiating benign lipoma from liposarcoma. Lesions deep to underlying fascia and those greater than 5 cm generally warrant further workup with tissue biopsy.[37] Core needle biopsy (CNB) performed under image guidance is the standard of care, demonstrating

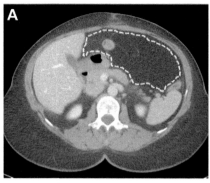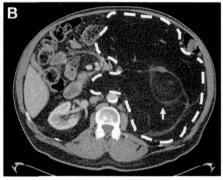

Fig. 3. CT of a retroperitoneal lipoma (*A*) and retroperitoneal WDLPS (*B*). Yellow dashed lines encircle tumor. Note that the tumors push the surrounding bowel and have low fat attenuation. The well-differentiated liposarcoma has thick septa (*arrow*), whereas the lipoma has fewer, thinner septa.

precision rates up to 98% in diagnosing benign from malignant lesions and accurately reflecting histology and grade in 75% and 80% of cases, respectively.[38,39] In a large cohort study of 530 patients undergoing CNB for suspected STM, only 7% of initial CNB were nondiagnostic and underwent repeat CNB.[39]

Smaller tumors less than 5 cm may be amenable to an excisional biopsy; however, when in doubt, it is best to pursue less invasive methods to obtain a tissue sample to avoid a scenario where positive excision margins complicate management. When a CNB or incisional biopsy is performed, the goal is to obtain an adequate tissue sample while minimizing contamination and avoiding the creation of hematoma/seroma via an approach that would not interfere with potential resection.[37] Specifically, biopsy needle tracts should be positioned such that they can be completely excised with the surgical specimen due to the potential seeding tumor along the tract.[40] This tends to be most important for larger extremity tumors in which orientation of the definitive surgical incision along the length of the extremity is needed. Pooled data from systematic reviews and case series suggest needle tract contamination (but not clinical recurrence) occurs in 13% and 0.37% extremity and retroperitoneal STS, respectively.[41–43] For this reason, some surgeons who perform resection of ALT/WDLPS prefer patients to be referred before biopsy of the lesion, so that the manner of biopsy can be directed by the operating surgeon. It should also be noted, particularly for retroperitoneal tumors where imaging is concordant with a lipoma or WDLPS, preoperative biopsy may not be clinically indicated before definitive surgical resection. This is because even with very large tumors, surgical resection represents the most effective treatment, there may be greater risk of injury to associated structures during biopsy, and often surgery is warranted regardless of the histologic diagnosis due to mass effect. If biopsy is undertaken, the trajectory of the biopsy needle should be aimed toward the most hyperenhancing and/or heterogeneous region of the tumor. This will help facilitate a diagnostic biopsy. Considered together, a good rule of thumb is if the initial treating physician does not intend to be the operative surgeon, discussion of biopsy or referral before biopsy for these types of tumors is warranted.

Histologically, simple lipomas are uniformly composed of mature adipocytes arranged in lobules surrounded by a thin fibrous capsule often without interdigitating septa (**Fig. 4**). ALT/WDLPS are more heterogenous masses that contain variably sized fats cells intermixed with scattered cells characterized by enlarged pleomorphic and hyperchromatic nuclei (**Fig. 5**). Fibrous septa are thicker, more abundant, and more

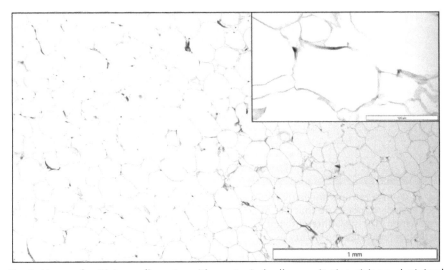

Fig. 4. Lipoma 4×. Mature adipocytes with no atypical cells, no mitotic activity, and minimal stroma. Insert: lipoma 40×. Mature adipocyte.

likely to enhance on contrast MRI of ALT/WDLPS compared with lipoma.[4] Low mitotic count, architectural disorganization, and the presence of adipocytic differentiation differentiates ALT/WDLPS from dedifferentiated LPS.[9] In contrast to much of the above evaluation, cytogenetic analysis demonstrates a stark distinction between lipoma and ALT/WDLPS—while both possess aberrations of chromosome 12q13 to 15, *MDM2* gene amplification, among others (**Table 3**), is seen in greater than 95% of ALT/WDLPS samples and absent in benign lipomas.[44,45] Although immunohistochemical staining and fluorescent in-situ hybridization (FISH) can both confirm amplification

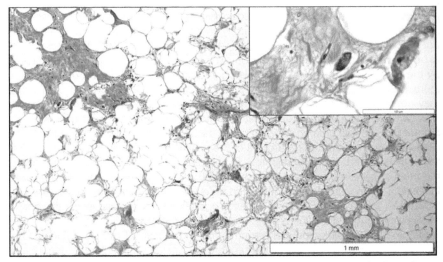

Fig. 5. WDLPS 4×. Mature adipocytes of varying size with scattered atypical cells with rare mitotic figures; fibrous stroma throughout. Insert: WDLPS 40×. Atypical cells with irregular nuclei within fibrous tissue.

Table 3
Biopsy, histologic, and molecular differences among lipoma, atypical lipomatous tumor, and well-differentiated liposarcomas[37,45]

	Lipoma	ALT	WDLPS
Biopsy considerations	Needle biopsy not generally needed; small lesions amenable to excisional biopsy	US guided; local anesthesia; 14–18G CNB; 4–10 passes; longitudinally oriented	CT vs US-guided; local anesthesia; ≥18G CNB; ≥6 passes; target nonfat or heterogenous component
Histologic findings	Mature adipocytes, encapsulating thin fibrous capsule; minimal septa	Variably sized adipocytes, pleomorphism, lipoblasts, and thick fibrous septa. Multiple histologic variants	
Molecular findings	12q15 rearrangement HMGA2 aberrations	12q13–15 amplification MDM2, CPM, HMGA2, CDK4, SAS amplification	

Abbreviations: CNB, core needle biopsy; CT, computed tomography; US, ultrasound.

of the *MDM2* gene, it should be noted that detection of *MDM2* gene amplification via FISH can take days or weeks longer to obtain. In most cases, a pathologist with experience in diagnosing mesenchymal tumors can accurately distinguish between these entities based on a review of standard hematoxylin and eosin (H&E)-stained sections.

Management

With a more definitive diagnosis in hand, supported by informed history and physical examination, appropriate imaging studies, and possible tissue diagnosis, therapeutic strategies can be devised. Based on this thorough workup, the practitioner should be guided by 1 of 3 scenarios—very likely/definitive benign adipocytic lesion (lipoma), very likely/definitive sarcoma, or lesion remains ambiguous. The latter two scenarios should be approached as a diagnosis of sarcoma. It is recommended that the definitive management of ALT/WDLPS occurs at high-volume sarcoma centers (defined as sarcoma referral centers or centers performing more than 20 cases per year) because registry-scale studies have demonstrated lower mortality rates, fewer positive margin resections, and decreased local recurrence rates at these centers.[46–48]

Staging

Unlike lipomas, formal oncologic staging of ALT/WDLPS should be performed. Staging is based on the American Joint Committee on Cancer (AJCC) TNM (Tumor, Node, Metastasis) system and tumor grade, the latter of which follows the French Federation of Cancer Centers Sarcoma Group scoring of tumor cell differentiation, mitotic activity, and extent of necrosis.[36] The need for additional imaging to complete staging should be considered. ALT generally does not require additional cross-sectional imaging given the extremely low risk of distant disease; however, if suspicious for high-grade components, chest imaging in chest X-ray or chest CT scan is warranted. Intraperitoneal/retroperitoneal WDLPS staging should include cross-sectional imaging of the chest despite the small, albeit not zero, chance of metastatic disease to the lungs.

Surgical excision

Local excision is the mainstay of treatment of symptomatic benign lipomas. Other indications include cosmesis and/or definitive tissue diagnosis generally in the setting of small tumors that can be resected without undue morbidity. Small, superficial extremity or truncal lesions often can be excised in the office setting under local anesthetic.[18] It is important to excise the lesion, maintaining the integrity of any tumor capsule to limit the risk of recurrence; wide margins are not necessary for lipomas unless suspicion for a more aggressive lesion is high. If, on final pathologic diagnosis, what was believed to be a benign lesion ultimately is found to be a STS with residual disease, salvage wide resection to obtain negative margins should be strongly considered if this can be performed without significantly increasing surgical morbidity.[49,50] Local recurrence rates are cited to be higher in these patients compared with those who undergo primary oncologic resection and/or unplanned excision with negative margins.[51–53] Re-excision for initially narrow but still negative margins is not generally indicated.

The cornerstone of treatment of ALT is surgical resection when possible. Complete resection is the best chance of cure as these are low-grade tumors with an incidence of histologic dedifferentiation ranging from 1% to 4%.[54] Wide resection (greater than 1 cm margin or intact fascial plane) with an attempt to include any biopsy tract to achieve negative margins is considered definitive resection by the National Cancer Center Network (NCCN).[36] As is often the case, ALT can abut and/or invade nearby structures such as bone, nerve, and vessels. Complete en bloc resection is not required if resection of adjacent critical structures would significantly increases surgical morbidity. Many surgeons will opt for a function preserving R1 resection (microscopically positive margins) with skeletonization of functionally important structures given the slow rate of growth and low risk of distant metastasis with recurrence. One large, single-center study of more than 800 patients with liposarcoma, 46% of whom had WDLPS, 12-year disease-specific survival (DSS) was not significantly different between negative resection margin (R0) and R1 resection.[13] A recent systematic review reported locoregional recurrence occurred in 12% of marginally resected ALT/WDLPS compared with 3% with wide excision; however, no impact on mortality with recurrence was noted and recurrences were typically amenable to low-morbidity re-resection.[55] Placement of titanium clips at the margins of an anticipated R1 resection can facilitate future surveillance and any other future locally directed therapies, such as radiation. Lymph node resection is not indicated in ALT or WDLPS because these tumors do not spread to lymph nodes.

Surgical wide resection is central to the treatment of retroperitoneal WDLPS and intra-abdominal lipomas. Although complete resection of the tumor with histologically clear margins is ideal, proximity to visceral structures and large size secondary to late presentation make complete resection or negative margins extremely challenging. The risks of the added morbidity must be weighed against microscopically negative margins. Residual disease is among the most important drivers of local recurrence as discussed in subsequent sections. Resection of all macroscopic disease without obligate resection of nearby structures is referred to as limited (or "marginal") resection and has been the dominant surgical approach because of the slow rate of growth and low risk of distant metastases with recurrence. Retroperitoneal structures that might be spared with this rationale include the kidney, ureter, bowel mesentery/blood supply, aorta, inferior vena cava, and the femoral nerve. Titanium clips again can be placed at the margins of an anticipated R1 resection to facilitate surveillance of local recurrence in the future.

In an effort to improve local control rates, sarcoma centers from France and Italy have recently advocated for extended resection, which involves en bloc removal of contiguous organs and structures that are not overtly involved, most commonly the kidney, ureter, colon, psoas muscle, and femoral nerve, citing decreased local recurrence rates with extended resection.[56,57] A recent retrospective, longer term analysis from a single-center suggests a statistically significant improvement in overall survival in addition to a trend toward improved local control specifically among low-grade liposarcomas (WDLPS and myxoid) undergoing extended resection.[57] In contrast, opponents of extended resection cite that nearly 70% of patients with initially unifocal WDLPS experience multifocal local recurrence, 18% of which is outside the original resection bed, questioning the necessity of resecting uninvolved organs and risking undue morbidity.[58] Functional status may be impacted with extended resection, particularly if the femoral nerve is sacrificed resulting in loss of hip flexion and knee extension. Nephrectomy results in a higher risk of developing end-stage renal disease.[59] Data from prospective trials comparing morbidity, quality of life measures, and long-term outcomes between the extended and limited/marginal resection are needed to clarify the optimal surgical approach.

Adjunct therapies
Direct injection of steroids into benign lipomas has been reported as an alternative to excision. One study examined prednisolone injection (0.07 mg) 5 days a week for 4 weeks—lipoma size decreased by 50%; however, by 1 year, 90% of lipomas increased in size and 80% of patients ultimately elected to have lesions excised.[60] Single-shot triamcinolone (40–80 mg) may be a more potent alternative associated with 60% reduction in lipoma volume at 4 months follow-up.[61] Intralesional steroid injection may be most appropriate for patients with small, symptomatic lesions averse to surgical excision or large lipomas warranting downsizing before excision; these indications must be considered in context of high failure rates and low-quality evidence supporting its use.

Neoadjuvant and adjuvant radiation therapy (RT) are well-studied adjuncts to the treatment of extremity liposarcoma. Before the acceptance of limb-sparing surgery, extremity amputation was the mainstay therapy for large, infiltrative extremity sarcomas. Not until the 1980 to 1990s did studies demonstrate no difference in overall survival between amputation versus wide resection with adjuvant RT, thus establishing limb-sparing surgery as the standard of care.[62,63] In a seminal analysis, Cassier and colleagues demonstrated a 74% reduction in local recurrence in those with ALT undergoing surgery with adjuvant RT versus surgery alone.[64] A 2018 meta-analysis of studies comparing surgery versus surgery plus external beam RT supported Cassier's findings that the latter group experienced decreased local recurrence across a variety of STSs of the head/neck, extremities, and trunk.[65] The most recent NCCN guidelines recommend considering RT for ALT with close margins without intact fascial plane where re-excision would result in functional morbidity.[36] When considering neoadjuvant versus adjuvant RT, acute wound complications associated with adjuvant therapy must be weighed against the larger required field, and long-term functional deficits attributed to limb edema, joint stiffness, and fibrosis associated with adjuvant RT.[66] As such, the decision to use RT should be made in a multidisciplinary setting (**Fig. 6**).

RT for retroperitoneal WDLPS is a contentious topic. Because complete macroscopic resection is achieved in less than 50% to 70% of patients, recurrence remains a significant burden. Early, nonrandomized, multi-institutional studies demonstrated a survival advantage to both adjuvant and neoadjuvant RT combined with surgery

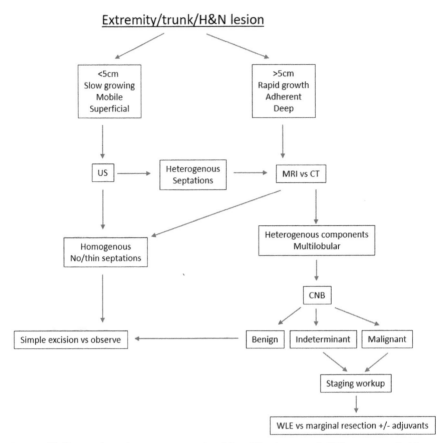

Fig. 6. ALT diagnostic and management algorithm. US, ultrasound; CNB, core needle biopsy; MRI, magnetic resonance imaging; CT, computed tomography.

compared with surgery alone.[67] However, results from the long-awaited randomized STRASS trial (Phase III Randomized Study of Preoperative Radiotherapy Plus Surgery vs Surgery Alone for Patients with Retroperitoneal Sarcoma: EORTC 62092) in which half of the patients received 50.4 Gy in 28 daily fractions 4 to 8 weeks preoperatively, failed to demonstrate improved abdominal-free recurrence survival or overall survival at a median follow-up of nearly 4 years.[68] In an unplanned post hoc analysis of only liposarcoma (75% of total cohort, including WDLPS and dedifferentiated liposarcoma), surgery with RT experienced a nonstatistically significant absolute improvement of 10% abdominal free recurrence compared with surgery alone at 3 years, suggesting there may be a role for RT in retroperitoneal LPS (75.7% vs 65.2%; HR 0.62, 95% CI 0.38–1.02). Nonetheless, the paucity of randomized trial data definitively supporting RT leaves the use of RT, preoperative or postoperative, heavily institution dependent; similar to ALT, the decision to use RT should be made in the multidisciplinary setting at high-volume sarcoma centers (**Fig. 7**).

ALT/WDLPS has minimal response to conventional chemotherapy with rates ranging from 0% to 12%.[69,70] In clinical practice, systemic chemotherapy is generally reserved for chemosensitive subtypes (eg, myxoid, synovial) and high-grade/AJCC stage II or greater lesions, which necessarily excludes low-grade ALT/WDLPS.[36]

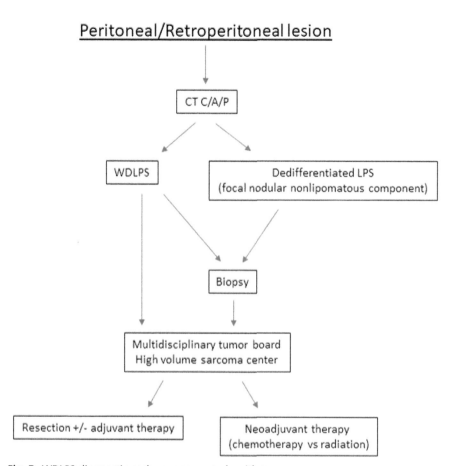

Fig. 7. WDLPS diagnostic and management algorithm.

Natural History, Surveillance, and Recurrence

Lipomas and ALT/WDLPS are slow-growing tumors. Lipomas and ALT have a mean time from symptom onset to presentation of 2 to 3 years.[20,71,72] After resection, lipomas and ALT have varying natural histories (**Table 4**). Benign, superficial lipomas have a reported recurrence rate of less than 5%.[4] In contrast, deep, intramuscular lipomas reportedly recur in 20% to 30% of cases, secondary to incomplete excision.[73] ALT has been cited to recur anywhere from 8% to 50%, a wide range stemming from variabilities in length of follow-up, resection margin status, and use of adjuvant therapies such as RT.[1,65,74,75] A recent analysis of 452 ALT, a majority of whom received R0 surgery alone, demonstrated local recurrence rate of 9.5% at 10 years.[76] The risk of local recurrence is greater for deep compared with superficial extremity/trunk tumors, sclerosing histologic subtype, intraoperative tumor rupture, and R1 resection.[75–78] In a large systematic review of ALT/WDLPS, local recurrence rates following marginal compared with wide resection were 11% vs 3%, respectively.[55] An analysis of 1000 patients with extremity or truncal STSs, 45% of whom had ALT, demonstrated that R1 resection was a significant predictor of local recurrence ($P = 0.002$, HR 2.3, CI 1.3–3.9).[76] Despite high local failure rates with R1 and marginal excision, neither DSS nor overall survival has been shown to be affected.[76,79] ALTs are slow-growing

Table 4
Treatment and long-term outcome differences among lipoma, atypical lipomatous tumor, and well-differentiated liposarcomas[36,76,84,87]

	Lipoma	ALT	WDLPS
Extent of surgery	Marginal	Marginal vs wide	Extended vs limited
Radiation	NA	Conditional	Conditional
Chemotherapy	NA	NA	NA
Local recurrence	1%–2%	8%–50% at 5 y	20%–90% at 5 y
Distant recurrence	NA	0.01% at 5 y	0.03% at 3 y
Overall survival	100%	>85% at 5 y	>77–90% at 5 y
Recommended surveillance	None	Physical examination with imaging Every 3–6 mo for first 2–3 y Annually thereafter	Physical examination with imaging Every 3–6 mo for first 2–3 y Every 6 mo for next 2 y Annually thereafter

tumors, with more than 75% of recurrences (following marginal and wide resections) occurring after 5 years postresection.[1,20,74,76] Reports of lipoma transformation to WDLPS, most commonly in the form of tumor recurrence, is rare, and suspect to histologic sampling error at the time of initial diagnosis of a benign lesion.[80] ALT does not have a propensity for metastatic disease unless it undergoes histologic dedifferentiation into a high-grade liposarcoma, which occurs in 1% to 5% of ALT.[10] Mortality has not been demonstrated to be different between lipomas and ALT. There is evidence that overall survival, but not disease-specific mortality, is decreased in ALT as compared with lipoma; this is because the median age of patients with ALT is generally greater than that of patients with lipomas.[81] Reported overall survival rates at 5 years for ALT are consistently greater than 85% to 90% with DSS nearing 100%.[2,16,82]

Compared with extremity/truncal lipomas and ALT, retroperitoneal WDLPS have higher recurrence and mortality rates. This is primarily due to the challenge of obtaining negative margins for large tumors with macro or microscopic involvement of adjacent structures. Causes of death from local recurrence frequently include bowel obstruction, renal failure, and severe malnutrition.[83] Local failure rates average 30% to 40% based on large-scale studies; however, rates as low as 5% and as high as 90% have been reported.[11,56,84,85] Similar to extremity STS studies, this wide range reflects the heterogenous composition of study populations, varying length of follow-up, and institution-dependent use of adjuvant therapies. Median time to recurrence ranges from 20 to 45 months.[85,86] In a study of 675 patients with retroperitoneal sarcoma, including 186 low-grade liposarcomas, predictors of local recurrence were age greater than 60 years ($P = 0.02$, HR 0.63, CI 0.5–0.8) and microscopically positive margins (compared with microscopically negative; $P < 0.01$, HR 1.5, CI 1.1–1.9).[87] In another study of 263 WDLPS, at 8 years follow-up, the local recurrence rate was 5% following extended resection with RT compared with 37% and 42% for those undergoing extended resection and limited resection alone, respectively.[85] For retroperitoneal liposarcomas at large, even microscopically positive resection margins significantly increase rate of abdominal recurrence.[56] Unlike extremity ALT, margin status is associated with survival in WDLPS as one study found DSS was 87%, 70%, and 43% with R0, R1, and R2 resections at 3 years, respectively ($P < 0.0001$).[13] Distant metastatic disease rarely, if ever, arises from primary WDLPS but rather occurs in setting of a local recurrence as the dedifferentiated subtype, a degeneration that occurs in 17% to 30% of WDLPS based on histopathologic analysis of recurrence resection specimens.[2,11] Each subsequent re-recurrence increases risk of dedifferentiation.[84] Overall survival at 5 years for WDLPS undergoing wide resection is 77% to 90%.[16,84,85]

Management of locally recurrent disease should be considered in a multidisciplinary setting at specialized sarcoma centers. Re-resection remains the mainstay of treatment of both extremity/abdominal wall and centrally located tumors. The morbidity of reoperation should be weighed against case-specific characteristics that contribute to prognosis such as recurrence location, surgical accessibility, and the surgical candidacy of the patient. One study found that resection of a surgically treatable local recurrence was associated with a survival of 53 months as compared with 30 months for patients who did not undergo surgery.[88] RT, alone or in combination with surgical resection, may be an option in select scenarios.[36]

Given the indolent biology yet high risk of local recurrence for ALT/WDLPS and the risk of dedifferentiation of WDLPS, long-term follow-up is recommended. Various sarcoma groups advocate follow-up durations ranging from 5 to 10 years.[75,89,90] NCCN guidelines suggest low-grade extremity/trunk tumors undergo clinic follow-up every 3 to 6 months in the first 2 to 3 years after resection, and annually after for at least 10 years in conjunction with baseline and interval imaging with MRI or CT of the primary site and chest to evaluate for metastases. For retroperitoneal lesions, recommended follow-up is every 3 to 6 months during the first 2 to 3 years postoperatively, then every 6 months for the next 2 years, then annually, in conjunction with cross-sectional imaging including the primary site and chest to evaluate for metastatic disease at these appointments.[36,76]

CLINICS CARE POINTS

- Ensure that the needle biopsy tract is included within planned surgical resection margins.

- Atypical lipomatous tumors (ALTs) are larger in size and have thicker and more abundant contrast-enhanced septa on magnetic resonance imaging.

- Intra-abdominal and retroperitoneal lipomatous masses cause intra-abdominal fullness and distention, are best evaluated by computed tomography, and are generally "pushing" rather than invading tumors.

- Benign lipomas should undergo marginal excision; when possible, wide resection should be attempted for ALT/well-differentiated liposarcomas.

- Long-term follow-up with interval cross-sectional imaging is imperative to identifying locoregional and distant recurrences.

DISCLOSURE

The authors have nothing to disclose.

REFERENCES

1. Kooby DA, Antonescu CR, Brennan MF, et al. Atypical lipomatous tumor/well-differentiated liposarcoma of the extremity and trunk wall: importance of histological subtype with treatment recommendations. Ann Surg Oncol 2004;11(1): 78–84.
2. Dalal KM, Antonescu CR, Singer S. Diagnosis and management of lipomatous tumors. J Surg Oncol 2008;97(4):298–313.

3. Bancroft LW, Kransdorf MJ, Peterson JJ, et al. Benign fatty tumors: classification, clinical course, imaging appearance, and treatment. Skeletal Radiol 2006;35(10): 719–33.
4. Murphey MD, Carroll JF, Flemming DJ, et al. From the archives of the AFIP: benign musculoskeletal lipomatous lesions. Radiographics 2004;24(5):1433–66.
5. Lowell A, Goldsmith SIK, Barbara A, et al. Chapter 129. Neoplasms of subcutaneous fat. *Fitzpatrick's Dermatology in general medicine*. New York City: McGraw-Hill, Medical Pub. Division; 2008. Chapter 129.
6. Aust MC, Spies M, Kall S, et al. Posttraumatic lipoma: fact or fiction? Skinmed 2007;6(6):266–70.
7. Signorini M, Campiglio GL. Posttraumatic lipomas: where do they really come from? Plast Reconstr Surg 1998;101(3):699–705.
8. WHO classification of tumours of soft tissue and bone. 5th edition. Lyon, FRANCE: IARC Press; 2021.
9. Lee ATJ, Thway K, Huang PH, et al. Clinical and molecular spectrum of liposarcoma. J Clin Oncol 2018;36(2):151–9.
10. Hogg ME, Wayne JD. Atypical lipomatous tumor/well-differentiated liposarcoma: what is it? Surg Oncol Clin N Am 2012;21(2):333–40.
11. Weiss SW, Rao VK. Well-differentiated liposarcoma (atypical lipoma) of deep soft tissue of the extremities, retroperitoneum, and miscellaneous sites. a follow-up study of 92 cases with analysis of the incidence of "dedifferentiation. Am J Surg Pathol 1992;16(11):1051–8.
12. Matthyssens LE, Creytens D, Ceelen WP. Retroperitoneal liposarcoma: current insights in diagnosis and treatment. Front Surg 2015;2:4.
13. Dalal KM, Kattan MW, Antonescu CR, et al. Subtype specific prognostic nomogram for patients with primary liposarcoma of the retroperitoneum, extremity, or trunk. Ann Surg 2006;244(3):381–91.
14. Mansfield SA, Pollock RE, Grignol VP. Surgery for abdominal well-differentiated liposarcoma. Curr Treat Options Oncol 2018;19(1):1.
15. Bock S, Hoffmann DG, Jiang Y, et al. Increasing incidence of liposarcoma: a population-based study of national surveillance databases, 2001-2016. Int J Environ Res Public Health 2020;17(8):2710.
16. Smith CA, Martinez SR, Tseng WH, et al. Predicting survival for well-differentiated liposarcoma: the importance of tumor location. J Surg Res 2012;175(1):12–7.
17. Bosetti C, La Vecchia C, Lipworth L, et al. Occupational exposure to vinyl chloride and cancer risk: a review of the epidemiologic literature. Eur J Cancer Prev 2003; 12(5):427–30.
18. Salam GA. Lipoma excision. Am Fam Physician 2002;65(5):901–4.
19. Rydholm A, Berg NO. Size, site and clinical incidence of lipoma. Factors in the differential diagnosis of lipoma and sarcoma. Acta Orthop Scand 1983;54(6): 929–34.
20. Rauh J, Klein A, Baur-Melnyk A, et al. The role of surgical margins in atypical lipomatous tumours of the extremities. BMC Musculoskelet Disord 2018;19(1):152.
21. Szewc M, Sitarz R, Moroz N, et al. Madelung's disease - progressive, excessive, and symmetrical deposition of adipose tissue in the subcutaneous layer: case report and literature review. Diabetes Metab Syndr Obes 2018;11:819–25.
22. Adiposa dolorosa. Available at. https://rarediseases.info.nih.gov/diseases/5750/adiposis-dolorosa. Accessed November 14, 2021.
23. Sachin Patil SS, Boram Ji, Ronald SC. Well-differentiated extremity and retroperitoneal liposarcoma: a population based outcome study. Surg Oncology Clin Pract J 2018;2(1).

24. Al-Ali MHM, Salih AM, Ahmed OF, et al. Retroperitoneal lipoma; a benign condition with frightening presentation. Int J Surg Case Rep 2019;57:63–6.
25. Kockerling F, Schug-Pass C. Spermatic cord lipoma-a review of the literature. Front Surg 2020;7:39.
26. Weniger M, D'Haese JG, Kunz W, et al. En-bloc resection of a giant retroperitoneal lipoma: a case report and review of the literature. BMC Res Notes 2015;8:75.
27. Murphey MD, Arcara LK, Fanburg-Smith J. From the archives of the AFIP: imaging of musculoskeletal liposarcoma with radiologic-pathologic correlation. Radiographics 2005;25(5):1371–95.
28. Roland CL. Soft tissue tumors of the extremity. Surg Clin North Am 2020;100(3): 669–80.
29. Kransdorf MJ, Bancroft LW, Peterson JJ, et al. Imaging of fatty tumors: distinction of lipoma and well-differentiated liposarcoma. Radiology 2002;224(1):99–104.
30. Ohguri T, Aoki T, Hisaoka M, et al. Differential diagnosis of benign peripheral lipoma from well-differentiated liposarcoma on MR imaging: is comparison of margins and internal characteristics useful? AJR Am J Roentgenol 2003;180(6): 1689–94.
31. Hosono M, Kobayashi H, Fujimoto R, et al. Septum-like structures in lipoma and liposarcoma: MR imaging and pathologic correlation. Skeletal Radiol 1997;26(3): 150–4.
32. Gaskin CM, Helms CA. Lipomas, lipoma variants, and well-differentiated liposarcomas (atypical lipomas): results of MRI evaluations of 126 consecutive fatty masses. AJR Am J Roentgenol 2004;182(3):733–9.
33. Panzarella MJ, Naqvi AH, Cohen HE, et al. Predictive value of gadolinium enhancement in differentiating ALT/WD liposarcomas from benign fatty tumors. Skeletal Radiol 2005;34(5):272–8.
34. Shaaban AM, Rezvani M, Tubay M, et al. Fat-containing retroperitoneal lesions: imaging characteristics, localization, and differential diagnosis. Radiographics 2016;36(3):710–34.
35. Messiou C, Morosi C. Imaging in retroperitoneal soft tissue sarcoma. J Surg Oncol 2018;117(1):25–32.
36. von Mehren M, Kane JM, Bui MM, et al. NCCN guidelines insights: soft tissue sarcoma, version 1.2021. J Natl Compr Canc Netw 2020;18(12):1604–12.
37. Tuttle R, Kane JM 3rd. Biopsy techniques for soft tissue and bowel sarcomas. J Surg Oncol 2015;111(5):504–12.
38. Heslin MJ, Lewis JJ, Woodruff JM, et al. Core needle biopsy for diagnosis of extremity soft tissue sarcoma. Ann Surg Oncol 1997;4(5):425–31.
39. Strauss DC, Qureshi YA, Hayes AJ, et al. The role of core needle biopsy in the diagnosis of suspected soft tissue tumours. J Surg Oncol 2010;102(5):523–9.
40. Schwartz HS, Spengler DM. Needle tract recurrences after closed biopsy for sarcoma: three cases and review of the literature. Ann Surg Oncol 1997;4(3):228–36.
41. Oliveira MP, Lima PM, da Silva HJ, et al. Neoplasm seeding in biopsy tract of the musculoskeletal system. a systematic review. Acta Ortop Bras 2014;22(2): 106–10.
42. UyBico SJ, Motamedi K, Omura MC, et al. Relevance of compartmental anatomic guidelines for biopsy of musculoskeletal tumors: retrospective review of 363 biopsies over a 6-year period. J Vasc Interv Radiol 2012;23(4):511–8.
43. Berger-Richardson D, Swallow CJ. Needle tract seeding after percutaneous biopsy of sarcoma: risk/benefit considerations. Cancer 2017;123(4):560–7.
44. Binh MB, Sastre-Garau X, Guillou L, et al. MDM2 and CDK4 immunostainings are useful adjuncts in diagnosing well-differentiated and dedifferentiated

liposarcoma subtypes: a comparative analysis of 559 soft tissue neoplasms with genetic data. Am J Surg Pathol 2005;29(10):1340–7.

45. Zhang H, Erickson-Johnson M, Wang X, et al. Molecular testing for lipomatous tumors: critical analysis and test recommendations based on the analysis of 405 extremity-based tumors. Am J Surg Pathol 2010;34(9):1304–11.

46. Gutierrez JC, Perez EA, Moffat FL, et al. Should soft tissue sarcomas be treated at high-volume centers? An analysis of 4205 patients. Ann Surg 2007;245(6):952–8.

47. Lazarides AL, Kerr DL, Nussbaum DP, et al. Soft Tissue Sarcoma of the Extremities: What Is the Value of Treating at High-volume Centers? Clin Orthop Relat Res 2019;477(4):718–27.

48. Blay JY, Honore C, Stoeckle E, et al. Surgery in reference centers improves survival of sarcoma patients: a nationwide study. Ann Oncol 2019;30(8):1407.

49. Bianchi G, Sambri A, Cammelli S, et al. Impact of residual disease after "unplanned excision" of primary localized adult soft tissue sarcoma of the extremities: evaluation of 452 cases at a single Institution. Musculoskelet Surg 2017; 101(3):243–8.

50. Charoenlap C, Imanishi J, Tanaka T, et al. Outcomes of unplanned sarcoma excision: impact of residual disease. Cancer Med 2016;5(6):980–8.

51. Ahlawat S, Fritz J, Morris CD, et al. Magnetic resonance imaging biomarkers in musculoskeletal soft tissue tumors: Review of conventional features and focus on nonmorphologic imaging. J Magn Reson Imaging 2019;50(1):11–27.

52. Qureshi YA, Huddy JR, Miller JD, et al. Unplanned excision of soft tissue sarcoma results in increased rates of local recurrence despite full further oncological treatment. Ann Surg Oncol 2012;19(3):871–7.

53. Liang Y, Guo TH, Xu BS, et al. The impact of unplanned excision on the outcomes of patients with soft tissue sarcoma of the trunk and extremity: a propensity score matching analysis. Front Oncol 2020;10:617590.

54. Nagano S, Yokouchi M, Setoguchi T, et al. Differentiation of lipoma and atypical lipomatous tumor by a scoring system: implication of increased vascularity on pathogenesis of liposarcoma. BMC Musculoskelet Disord 2015;16:36.

55. Choi KY, Jost E, Mack L, et al. Surgical management of truncal and extremities atypical lipomatous tumors/well-differentiated liposarcoma: A systematic review of the literature. Am J Surg 2020;219(5):823–7.

56. Bonvalot S, Rivoire M, Castaing M, et al. Primary retroperitoneal sarcomas: a multivariate analysis of surgical factors associated with local control. J Clin Oncol 2009;27(1):31–7.

57. Gronchi A, Miceli R, Colombo C, et al. Frontline extended surgery is associated with improved survival in retroperitoneal low- to intermediate-grade soft tissue sarcomas. Ann Oncol 2012;23(4):1067–73.

58. Tseng WW, Madewell JE, Wei W, et al. Locoregional disease patterns in well-differentiated and dedifferentiated retroperitoneal liposarcoma: implications for the extent of resection? Ann Surg Oncol 2014;21(7):2136–43.

59. Ellis RJ. Chronic kidney disease after nephrectomy: a clinically-significant entity? Transl Androl Urol 2019;8(Suppl 2):S166–74.

60. Redman LM, Moro C, Dobak J, et al. Association of beta-2 adrenergic agonist and corticosteroid injection in the treatment of lipomas. Diabetes Obes Metab 2011;13(6):517–22.

61. Hayward WA, Sibbitt WL, Sibbitt RR, et al. Intralesional Injection of Triamcinolone Acetonide for Subcutaneous Lipoma causing Musculoskeletal and Neurologic Symptoms. J Clin Aesthet Dermatol 2018;11(5):38–42.

62. Rosenberg SA, Tepper J, Glatstein E, et al. The treatment of soft-tissue sarcomas of the extremities: prospective randomized evaluations of (1) limb-sparing surgery plus radiation therapy compared with amputation and (2) the role of adjuvant chemotherapy. Ann Surg 1982;196(3):305–15.

63. Baldini EH, Goldberg J, Jenner C, et al. Long-term outcomes after function-sparing surgery without radiotherapy for soft tissue sarcoma of the extremities and trunk. J Clin Oncol 1999;17(10):3252–9.

64. Cassier PA, Kantor G, Bonvalot S, et al. Adjuvant radiotherapy for extremity and trunk wall atypical lipomatous tumor/well-differentiated LPS (ALT/WD-LPS): a French Sarcoma Group (GSF-GETO) study. Ann Oncol 2014;25(9):1854–60.

65. Albertsmeier M, Rauch A, Roeder F, et al. External beam radiation therapy for resectable soft tissue sarcoma: a systematic review and meta-analysis. Ann Surg Oncol 2018;25(3):754–67.

66. Gamboa AC, Gronchi A, Cardona K. Soft-tissue sarcoma in adults: An update on the current state of histiotype-specific management in an era of personalized medicine. CA Cancer J Clin 2020;70(3):200–29.

67. Nussbaum DP, Rushing CN, Lane WO, et al. Preoperative or postoperative radiotherapy versus surgery alone for retroperitoneal sarcoma: a case-control, propensity score-matched analysis of a nationwide clinical oncology database. Lancet Oncol 2016;17(7):966–75.

68. Bonvalot S, Gronchi A, Le Pechoux C, et al. Preoperative radiotherapy plus surgery versus surgery alone for patients with primary retroperitoneal sarcoma (EORTC-62092: STRASS): a multicentre, open-label, randomised, phase 3 trial. Lancet Oncol 2020;21(10):1366–77.

69. Jones RL, Fisher C, Al-Muderis O, et al. Differential sensitivity of liposarcoma subtypes to chemotherapy. Eur J Cancer 2005;41(18):2853–60.

70. Italiano A, Toulmonde M, Cioffi A, et al. Advanced well-differentiated/dedifferentiated liposarcomas: role of chemotherapy and survival. Ann Oncol 2012;23(6):1601–7.

71. Fisher SB, Baxter KJ, Staley CA 3rd, et al. The general surgeon's quandary: atypical lipomatous tumor vs lipoma, who needs a surgical oncologist? J Am Coll Surg 2013;217(5):881–8.

72. Yamamoto N, Hayashi K, Tanzawa Y, et al. Treatment strategies for well-differentiated liposarcomas and therapeutic outcomes. Anticancer Res 2012; 32(5):1821–5.

73. Hornick J. Practical soft tissue pathology: a diagnostic approach. 2nd edition. Philadelphia, PA: Elsevier; 2019.

74. Evans HL. Atypical lipomatous tumor, its variants, and its combined forms: a study of 61 cases, with a minimum follow-up of 10 years. Am J Surg Pathol 2007;31(1):1–14.

75. Rozental TD, Khoury LD, Donthineni-Rao R, et al. Atypical lipomatous masses of the extremities: outcome of surgical treatment. Clin Orthop Relat Res 2002;398: 203–11.

76. Bartlett EK, Curtin CE, Seier K, et al. Histologic subtype defines the risk and kinetics of recurrence and death for primary extremity/truncal liposarcoma. Ann Surg 2021;273(6):1189–96.

77. Lucas DR, Nascimento AG, Sanjay BK, et al. Well-differentiated liposarcoma. the mayo clinic experience with 58 cases. Am J Clin Pathol 1994;102(5):677–83.

78. Mussi CE, Daolio P, Cimino M, et al. Atypical lipomatous tumors: should they be treated like other sarcoma or not? Surgical consideration from a bi-institutional experience. Ann Surg Oncol 2014;21(13):4090–7.

79. Bonvalot S, Levy A, Terrier P, et al. Primary extremity soft tissue sarcomas: does local control impact survival? Ann Surg Oncol 2017;24(1):194–201.
80. Lee YJ, Cha WJ, Kim Y, et al. The recurrence of well-differentiated liposarcoma from benign giant intramuscular lipoma: A case (CARE-compliant) report. Medicine (Baltimore) 2021;100(6):e24711.
81. Presman B, Jauffred SF, Korno MR, et al. Low recurrence rate and risk of distant metastases following marginal surgery of intramuscular lipoma and atypical lipomatous tumors of the extremities and trunk wall. Med Princ Pract 2020;29(3):203–10.
82. Vos M, Kosela-Paterczyk H, Rutkowski P, et al. Differences in recurrence and survival of extremity liposarcoma subtypes. Eur J Surg Oncol 2018;44(9):1391–7.
83. Canter RJ, Qin LX, Ferrone CR, et al. Why do patients with low-grade soft tissue sarcoma die? Ann Surg Oncol 2008;15(12):3550–60.
84. Singer S, Antonescu CR, Riedel E, et al. Histologic subtype and margin of resection predict pattern of recurrence and survival for retroperitoneal liposarcoma. Ann Surg 2003;238(3):358–70 ; discussion 370-1.
85. Gronchi A, Strauss DC, Miceli R, et al. Variability in patterns of recurrence after resection of primary retroperitoneal sarcoma (RPS): a report on 1007 patients from the multi-institutional collaborative RPS working group. Ann Surg 2016;263(5):1002–9.
86. Knebel C, Lenze U, Pohlig F, et al. Prognostic factors and outcome of Liposarcoma patients: a retrospective evaluation over 15 years. BMC Cancer 2017;17(1):410.
87. Tan MC, Brennan MF, Kuk D, et al. Histology-based classification predicts pattern of recurrence and improves risk stratification in primary retroperitoneal sarcoma. Ann Surg 2016;263(3):593–600.
88. Lochan R, French JJ, Manas DM. Surgery for retroperitoneal soft tissue sarcomas: aggressive re-resection of recurrent disease is possible. Ann R Coll Surg Engl 2011;93(1):39–43.
89. Kito M, Yoshimura Y, Isobe K, et al. Clinical outcome of deep-seated atypical lipomatous tumor of the extremities with median-term follow-up study. Eur J Surg Oncol 2015;41(3):400–6.
90. Sommerville SM, Patton JT, Luscombe JC, et al. Clinical outcomes of deep atypical lipomas (well-differentiated lipoma-like liposarcomas) of the extremities. ANZ J Surg 2005;75(9):803–6.

Dermatofibrosarcoma Protuberans: What Is This?

Gerardo A. Vitiello, MD[a], Ann Y. Lee, MD[a,b], Russell S. Berman, MD[a,b,*]

KEYWORDS

• Dermatofibrosarcoma protuberans • DFSP • Surgical considerations

KEY POINTS

• Dermatofibrosarcoma (DFSP) may be misinterpreted as a clinically benign lesion, leading to inadequate surgical excision.
• Negative margin surgical resection is the potentially curative treatment of DFSP.
• Fibrosarcomatous transformation is associated with increased metastatic potential and should be managed in a multidisciplinary fashion, including the consideration of adjuvant therapy and clinical trials.
• In the setting of an extensive resection, reconstruction should be delayed until a definitive pathologic margin assessment to minimize recurrence.

NATURE OF THE PROBLEM

Dermatofibrosarcoma protuberans (DFSP) is a rare, dermal-based sarcoma that, in the absence of fibrosarcomatous transformation, has an extremely low metastatic potential, but exhibits highly aggressive tissue infiltration with a proclivity for local recurrence. The most effective primary treatment is negative margin surgical resection. Given its locally aggressive nature, obtaining pathologically negative margins at the index operation is critical to improving recurrence-free survival.

Unfortunately, DFSP can clinically mimic benign neoplasms such as a dermatofibroma, keloid, lipoma, or abscess. As a result, diagnosis is often delayed, especially when the clinical suspicion is low. Perhaps more challenging is the fact that diagnosis may often be discovered incidentally after surgical resection for what was thought to be a benign lesion. In these scenarios, surgical margins are likely to be inadequate and local recurrence is likely. In this article, DFSP as a diagnostic consideration even for

[a] Department of Surgery, Division of Surgical Oncology, New York University Langone Health, 550 First Avenue, NBV 15 North-1, New York, NY 10016, USA; [b] Department of Surgery, Surgical Residency and Education Program, NYU Grossman School of Medicine, 160 East 34th Street, 7th Floor, New York, NY 10016, USA
* Corresponding author. Surgical Residency Program, Division of Surgical Oncology, NYU Grossman School of Medicine, 160 East 34th Street, 7th Floor, New York, NY 10016, USA.
E-mail address: Russell.Berman@nyulangone.org
Twitter: @GerardoVitiello (G.A.V.); @AnnYLeeSurgOnc (A.Y.L.); @bermar01 (R.S.B.)

Surg Clin N Am 102 (2022) 657–665
https://doi.org/10.1016/j.suc.2022.05.004   surgical.theclinics.com
0039-6109/22/© 2022 Elsevier Inc. All rights reserved.

what may seem to be a clinically benign lesion will be emphasized. The workup, surgical management, and surveillance for this challenging entity will also be discussed.

BACKGROUND AND CLINICAL CONSIDERATIONS

Although rare, DFSP is one of the most common dermal sarcomas with an incidence of approximately 4.2 cases per million people in the United States.[1] DFSP represents 18% of cutaneous soft tissue sarcomas and typically occurs in the third to fifth decades of life.[2] Males are 1.14 times more likely to be affected versus women, and African Americans are twice as likely to develop a DFSP as compared with Caucasians.[3] DFSP is most frequently identified on the trunk (42%), followed by the upper and lower extremities (41%), and head and neck (16%), particularly on the scalp, supraclavicular fossa, and forehead.[1,4,5] While the etiology and clinical risk factors have not been completely elucidated, DFSP has been reported to be associated with sites of prior trauma or scar.[6,7]

Often progressing slowly over years, DFSP typically presents as a painless, indurated plaque or mass with a violaceous, pink, or reddish-brown appearance (**Fig. 1**A). Although it often starts as a single lesion, satellite nodules can develop and help to distinguish a DFSP from other pathologic entities. DFSP is frequently firm to palpation and is usually fixed within the dermis, but not necessarily the underlying subcutaneous tissues. Given that DFSP can have irregular borders and fingerlike extensions into the deeper tissue, clinical examination should focus on the visual and palpable extent of disease with additional attention to possible fixation to deep structures and the presence of any satellite nodules. If DFSP is suspected, the clinical assessment should also take into consideration surgical resection and reconstructive options. Although less than 5% of patients will develop nodal or distant metastatic disease,[8] a regional lymph node examination should be performed, especially if the diagnosis of DFSP has not yet been confirmed.

Imaging evaluation is not required for small lesions, but it may assist in the surgical planning of larger lesions. In particular, imaging can help to determine the depth of invasion. Per NCCN guidelines, contrast-enhanced MRI is the preferred diagnostic modality in the workup of DFSP to assess for tissue involvement and depth.[9] A tissue diagnosis is indicated if DFSP is suspected. A core needle or punch biopsy is

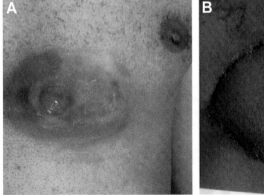
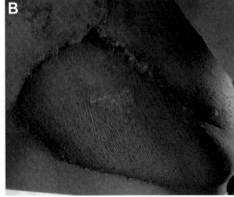

Fig. 1. Primary, chest wall DFSP. (*A*) Preoperative photo of primary chest wall DFSP mistakenly diagnosed as chest wall abscess. Central area of ulceration is secondary to incision and drainage attempts. (*B*) Postresection photo with full-thickness skin graft.

preferred over an incisional biopsy. NCCN guidelines recommend that mitotic rate and the presence or absence of fibrosarcomatous transformation should be noted in a DFSP biopsy pathology report.[10]

PATHOLOGIC EVALUATION AND GENETICS

Histologically, DFSP is a dermal-based tumor characterized by a dense proliferation of uniform spindle cells with limited pleomorphism and low mitotic activity.[5] Most of DFSP (80%–100%) stain positive for the mesenchymal cell marker CD34 and vimentin,[5] while negative for factor XIIIA, desmin, smooth muscle actin, S100, and keratin. Appropriate immunohistochemical staining should be performed on all suspected DFSP specimens.

Most cases of DFSP are characterized by a supernumerary ring chromosome that leads to reciprocal translocation t(17;22) (q22;q13) and a fusion between platelet-derived growth factor B-chain (PDGFB) and collagen type 1 alpha 1 (COL1A1) genes.[11,12] In fact, the COL1A1-PDGFB fusion gene has been identified in nearly 85% to 95% of tumors. Reverse transcriptase polymerase chain reaction has allowed for a more accurate evaluation of the cytogenetic rearrangements in DFSP, which has important implications for targeted molecular therapy with tyrosine kinase inhibitors.

There are multiple subtypes of DFSP, including giant cell fibroblastoma, pigmented (Bednar), atrophic, sclerosing, myxoid, myoid, granular cell, and fibrosarcomatous transformation, each having a characteristic histologic appearance for which it is named. Clinically, most subtypes are associated with a recurrence risk of 20% to 50% with the exception of Bednar (which has a low 11%–13% recurrence rate) and fibrosarcomatous transformation (which has a somewhat high 55% recurrence risk).[13]

Although DFSP with fibrosarcomatous transformation (DFSP-FS) has the same characteristic chromosomal rearrangements, it is typically considered a true sarcoma and is distinguished from DFSP by cytologic atypia, increased cellularity, increased mitotic activity, and lack of CD34 expression.[14] Moreover, metastases can occur in up to 14% of DFSP-FS cases.[15] As a result, the presence of DFSP-FS on biopsy should be managed as a true sarcoma in a multidisciplinary fashion, including consideration for adjuvant therapy and clinical trials.

MANAGEMENT CONSIDERATIONS

Increased tumor size and depth are associated with a higher risk of subclinical extension and local recurrence. Therefore, these are important considerations when choosing a surgical approach. One study showed that deep tumors, defined as extending to the fascia directly beneath the primary lesion, were associated with an increased risk for local recurrence (HR 3.14, 95% CI [1.18–8.32]).[16] The potentially curative treatment of DFSP is negative margin surgical resection. Mohs micrographic surgery (MMS) has also been used as a real-time margin assessment surgical approach for the treatment of DFSP. However, no prospective, randomized clinical trials have been performed showing the superiority of MMS over conventional surgical resection.[4] Although one systematic review of retrospective studies did show lower local recurrence rates for MMS versus wide resection,[17] limitations include fairly short follow-ups and a potential bias toward the use of MMS for smaller, lower risk tumors.

Based on multiple large, population-based studies totaling nearly 10,000 patients, overall survival for DFSP is excellent, approaching 100% at 15 years.[1,3] However, local recurrence is a significant issue as nearly 13% of primary DFSPs will recur after initial treatment. In addition, 33% of patients with recurrent DFSP treated with surgical resection experienced an additional recurrence.[16] Prognostic factors associated with a decreased overall survival include advanced age at diagnosis, black race, male gender, head or limb tumor location, tumor size, and fibrosarcomatous transformation.[13,18] Risk factors associated with a worse recurrence-free survival include tumor depth, margin status, fibrosarcomatous change, increased cellularity, high mitotic rate, and patient age over 50.[16,19] In a retrospective series of 67 patients with DFSP, 5 patients went on to develop metastatic disease; 4 of the 5 (80%) had a primary tumor size larger than 10 cm, suggesting that larger tumor size is associated with increased metastasis risk.[20]

Procedural Approach

As previously noted, the first attempt at surgical resection has the greatest impact on the recurrence-free survival of DFSP. One of the defining characteristics of DFSP is long, irregular, subclinical, and tentacle-like extensions into the subcutaneous fat. In fact, extension is unpredictable and can vary from 0.3 cm to 12 cm beyond the macroscopic borders.[8,21] Whether approached by Moh's micrographic surgery or by standard surgical resection, every effort should be made to achieve negative surgical margins and some form of complete histologic surgical margin assessment is strongly recommended.[10] In general, the surgeon should avoid undermining tissue planes, which can complicate margin assessment.[22] Transverse incisions along the extremity should be avoided for both the biopsy and the definitive resection as it will limit reconstructive options, especially if reresection is required.

Radial Margins

The clinical resection margin is strongly correlated with the risk of local recurrence. It has been shown that 1 cm margins around the primary tumor leave residual microscopic tumor in approximately 70% of patients; 2 cm margins in 20% to 40% of patients, 3 cm in 9% to 16% of patients, and 5 cm in 5% of patients.[21,23,24] While 5 cm margins may result in the lowest risk of recurrence, the surgeon must weigh a high rate of local control against the functional and cosmetic impact of the large soft tissue defect created. In one study of more than 200 patients with DFSP, margins of at least 2 cm were associated with a recurrence rate of less than 1%.[25] As a result, the NCCN recommends 2 cm margins in the surgical resection of DFSP.[9]

Deep Margins

In addition to 2 cm radial margins, a microscopically negative deep margin is also necessary. Fields and colleagues have suggested removing the underlying muscular fascia to eliminate deeply infiltrating cells, as tumor depth is independently associated with recurrence-free survival.[16] As previously discussed, cross-sectional imaging (preferably MRI with and without intravenous contrast) will help plan the deep extent of resection and should be obtained for any lesion that is not clinically superficial. Fascia, periosteum, and/or cartilage at the deep margin should be resected en-bloc with the specimen to maximize the chance of an R0 (microscopic negative margin) resection. In a study of MMS for DFSP, 17/40 patients (43%) required fascia, muscle, or periosteal resection to obtain tumor clearance.[26]

Intraoperative Margin Assessment

If considering intraoperative margin assessment. intraoperative frozen section can be unreliable with false-negative rates as high as 57%.[27] While a positive frozen section might be beneficial in certain situations to aid in resecting more tissue at that particular location, negative results in frozen section should be interpreted with caution and must not be considered definitive. When complex tissue reconstruction is required after resection, it is prudent to consider a temporary dressing and delayed reconstruction while awaiting the final pathologic margin assessment.

Staged Surgical Resections with En Face Margin Assessment

Given that the unique expertise necessary for MMS is not available at all institutions, a similar alternative approach using more traditional surgery would be staged surgical resections with en face pathologic margin assessment ("slow Mohs"). The initial surgical resection could be planned with more limited margins (1–2 cm). Before resection, both the margins of the specimen as well as the surrounding native tissues are precisely marked in a clock face manner (12:00, 3:00, 6:00, and so forth) for future identification. Following the first stage of resection, the specimen is carefully oriented for pathology to exactly correspond to the specific locations marked at the resection edges within the patient. The resection defect is left open pending margin confirmation. As opposed to the more traditional tangential margin assessment (that typically evaluates only a small percentage of the total margin), en face margin assessment by pathology will assess 100% of the margin, including the deep margin. In contrast to intraoperative frozen section, staged surgeries with delayed reconstruction also allow pathology to do a more definitive margin assessment, including immunohistochemistry. Based on the precise orientation, pathology can identify specific areas of residual DFSP at the margin (eg, 2–3 o'clock). Additional staged resections can then be performed only at the location of the positive margins. As with MMS, although staged resections may require several surgeries to clear specific margins with persistent DFSP, this will result in the smallest possible surgical defect with pathologically confirmed 100% negative margins. Once all margins are negative, definitive closure of the surgical defect can be performed.

Reconstruction

As previously stated, delayed reconstruction is recommended in cases requiring extensive resection or tissue manipulation. This will allow for the confirmation of negative pathologic margins before undertaking a reconstruction. Negative pressure therapy can be helpful while awaiting final margin status and reconstructive consultation is recommended.[28] Rotational flaps and full- or split-thickness skin grafts (**Fig. 1**B) are all options. The choice of reconstruction is multifactorial, based on factors such as size, depth, and location of the surgical defect. In the event that negative microscopic margins are not achievable, skin grafts generally simplify monitoring for local recurrence.

Recurrent and Residual Dermatofibrosarcoma Protuberans

Recurrent DFSP is managed similarly to primary DFSP; resection to negative radial and deep margins with delayed reconstruction until the final pathology confirms negative margins (**Fig. 2**). In regard to residual DFSP following prior resection, if there are positive margins after the initial resection, reresection should be considered if it is technically possible to achieve negative margins and additional surgery would not result in significant functional deficits or operative morbidity.

Radiation Therapy

Although several studies have shown that adjuvant radiation therapy can reduce local recurrence in patients with DFSP with close or positive margins (10-year local control rates up to 88%),[13,29–31] a recent meta-analysis by Chen and colleagues found no statistical difference in recurrence rates between surgery alone and surgery with adjuvant radiation.[32] Therefore, adjuvant radiation is not currently recommended in the setting of margin negative resection.[9] However, adjuvant radiation can be considered in

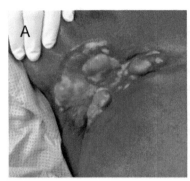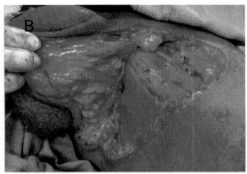

Fig. 2. Recurrent, groin DFSP. (*A*) Preoperative photo of recurrent DFSP, multilobulated in appearance. (*B*) Postresection photo. Note that the fascia of the adductor muscle has been resected, with plans for the application of a vacuum-assisted wound closure dressing before final pathology result and reconstruction.

cases of R1 resection whereby attempting an R0 reresection would result in significant functional, cosmetic, or operative morbidity. Doses of 50 to 60 Gy for indeterminate or positive margins and up to 66 Gy for gross residual tumor are used with fields extending widely beyond the surgical margin when feasible. Given the lack of consensus in the literature, these cases should be discussed at a multidisciplinary tumor board with an individualized plan developed for each patient.

Systemic Therapy

Conventional cytotoxic chemotherapy has generally been ineffective for DFSP and currently has a minimal role in treatment. The COL1A1-PDGFB fusion protein (identified in nearly 85%–95% of DFSPs) resulting in activated PDGFB signaling has led to the use of tyrosine kinase inhibitors for the treatment of DFSP. For patients with DFSP with locally advanced or metastatic disease, tyrosine kinase inhibitors have produced response rates of 50% to 60%.[33] One phase II trial demonstrated a 36% clinical response rate in patients treated with neoadjuvant imatinib,[34] while another phase II DeCOG trial showed a response rate of 57%.[35] As a result, imatinib has also been FDA approved for the treatment of unresectable, recurrent, and/or metastatic DFSP.[36] Sunitinib, another tyrosine kinase inhibitor, had a 40% response rate in patients with imatinib-resistant DFSP.[37] Other tyrosine kinase inhibitors, including sorafenib and pazopanib, have been effective in smaller studies or case reports.[38,39]

FOLLOW-UP AND SURVEILLANCE

Patients with DFSP require long-term follow-up. Local recurrences are common and can occur greater than 5 years from initial surgery.[17] The decision of whether to follow patients with clinical examination alone versus cross-sectional imaging depends on the initial size, depth, and location of the primary tumor as well as the type of reconstruction used. For large, deep-seated tumors, complex reconstructions, or multiple recurrences that make physical examination difficult to interpret, surveillance MRI can provide additional information. Although metastatic disease is not common with DFSP, patients with DFSP-FS should undergo chest imaging as per the NCCN guidelines for soft tissue sarcomas.

SUMMARY

Dermatofibrosarcoma protuberans is a rare, dermal-based sarcoma with a very low metastatic potential in the absence of fibrosarcomatous transformation, but an infiltrative growth pattern associated with high rates of local recurrence. The presence of fibrosarcomatous transformation increases metastatic risk and warrants treatment as a true sarcoma. MMS, wide surgical resection with at least 2 cm margins, or staged surgical resections with en face margin assessment are all surgical options for DFSP to increase the likelihood of a negative margin resection on final pathology. Delayed reconstruction for large surgical defects that require complex reconstruction and tissue rearrangement for wound coverage is recommended. Adjuvant radiation can reduce the risk of local recurrence in patients with positive margins whereby additional resection would result in significant functional or cosmetic morbidity. The characteristic fusion gene COL1A1-PDGFB makes tyrosine kinase inhibitors such as imatinib a potential treatment option for locally advanced, recurrent, or metastatic DFSP.

CLINICS CARE POINTS

- A biopsy should be performed for all suspected DFSP, including the presence or absence of fibrosarcomatous change and mitotic rate on the pathology report.
- The presence of fibrosarcomatous change warrants management as a true fibrosarcoma.
- Surgical resection with negative margins is the mainstay of DFSP treatment. Following an extensive resection, reconstruction should be delayed until definitive pathologic margin assessment is available.
- Radiation can have a role to reduce local recurrence with positive margins when reresection would result in significant morbidity.
- Tyrosine kinase inhibitors may delay progression in unresectable or metastatic disease.

DISCLOSURE

The authors have declared that no conflicts of interest exist.

REFERENCES

1. Criscione VD, Weinstock MA. Descriptive epidemiology of dermatofibrosarcoma protuberans in the United States, 1973 to 2002. J Am Acad Dermatol 2007;56(6): 968–73.
2. Rouhani P, Fletcher CDM, Devesa SS, et al. Cutaneous soft tissue sarcoma incidence patterns in the U.S. : an analysis of 12,114 cases. Cancer 2008;113(3): 616–27.
3. Kreicher KL, Kurlander DE, Gittleman HR, et al. Incidence and Survival of Primary Dermatofibrosarcoma Protuberans in the United States. Dermatol Surg 2016; 42(Suppl 1):S24–31.
4. Acosta AE, Velez CS. Dermatofibrosarcoma Protuberans. Curr Treat Options Oncol 2017;18(9):56.
5. Llombart B, Serra C, Requena C, et al. Guidelines for Diagnosis and Treatment of Cutaneous Sarcomas: Dermatofibrosarcoma Protuberans. Actas Dermosifiliogr 2018;109(10):868–77.
6. McPeak CJ, Cruz T, Nicastri AD. Dermatofibrosarcoma protuberans: an analysis of 86 cases–five with metastasis. Ann Surg 1967;166(5):803–16.

7. Kneebone RL, Melissas J, Mannell A. Dermatofibrosarcoma protuberans in black patients. S Afr Med J 1984;66(24):919–21.

8. Allen A, Ahn C, Sangüeza OP. Dermatofibrosarcoma Protuberans. Dermatol Clin 2019;37(4):483–8.

9. Bichakjian CK, Olencki T, Alam M, et al. Dermatofibrosarcoma protuberans, version 1.2014. J Natl Compr Canc Netw 2014 Jun;12(6):863–8. https://doi.org/10.6004/jnccn.2014.0081. PMID: 24925197.

10. Miller SJ, Alam M, Andersen JS, et al. Dermatofibrosarcoma protuberans. J Natl Compr Canc Netw 2012;10(3):312–8.

11. Mandahl N, Heim S, Willén H, et al. Supernumerary ring chromosome as the sole cytogenetic abnormality in a dermatofibrosarcoma protuberans. Cancer Genet Cytogenet 1990;49(2):273–5.

12. Simon MP, Pedeutour F, Sirvent N, et al. Deregulation of the platelet-derived growth factor B-chain gene via fusion with collagen gene COL1A1 in dermatofibrosarcoma protuberans and giant-cell fibroblastoma. Nat Genet 1997;15(1):95–8.

13. Iwasaki T, Yamamoto H, Oda Y. Current Update on the Molecular Biology of Cutaneous Sarcoma: Dermatofibrosarcoma Protuberans. Curr Treat Options Oncol 2019;20(4):29.

14. Palmerini E, Gambarotti M, Staals EL, et al. Fibrosarcomatous changes and expression of CD34+ and apolipoprotein-D in dermatofibrosarcoma protuberans. Clin Sarcoma Res 2012;2(1):4.

15. Mentzel T, Beham A, Katenkamp D, et al. Fibrosarcomatous ("high-grade") dermatofibrosarcoma protuberans: clinicopathologic and immunohistochemical study of a series of 41 cases with emphasis on prognostic significance. Am J Surg Pathol 1998;22(5):576–87.

16. Fields RC, Hameed M, Qin L-X, et al. Dermatofibrosarcoma protuberans (DFSP): predictors of recurrence and the use of systemic therapy. Ann Surg Oncol 2011;18(2):328–36.

17. Foroozan M, Sei J-F, Amini M, et al. Efficacy of Mohs micrographic surgery for the treatment of dermatofibrosarcoma protuberans: systematic review. Arch Dermatol 2012;148(9):1055–63.

18. Criscito MC, Martires KJ, Stein JA. Prognostic Factors, Treatment, and Survival in Dermatofibrosarcoma Protuberans. JAMA Dermatol 2016;152(12):1365–71.

19. Bowne WB, Antonescu CR, Leung DH, et al. Dermatofibrosarcoma protuberans: A clinicopathologic analysis of patients treated and followed at a single institution. Cancer 2000;88(12):2711–20.

20. Hayakawa K, Matsumoto S, Ae K, et al. Risk factors for distant metastasis of dermatofibrosarcoma protuberans. J Orthop Traumatol 2016;17(3):261–6.

21. Ratner D, Thomas CO, Johnson TM, et al. Mohs micrographic surgery for the treatment of dermatofibrosarcoma protuberans. Results of a multiinstitutional series with an analysis of the extent of microscopic spread. J Am Acad Dermatol 1997;37(4):600–13.

22. DuBay D, Cimmino V, Lowe L, et al. Low recurrence rate after surgery for dermatofibrosarcoma protuberans: a multidisciplinary approach from a single institution. Cancer 2004;100(5):1008–16.

23. Loghdey MS, Varma S, Rajpara SM, et al. Mohs micrographic surgery for dermatofibrosarcoma protuberans (DFSP): a single-centre series of 76 patients treated by frozen-section Mohs micrographic surgery with a review of the literature. J Plast Reconstr Aesthet Surg 2014;67(10):1315–21.

24. Parker TL, Zitelli JA. Surgical margins for excision of dermatofibrosarcoma protuberans. J Am Acad Dermatol 1995;32(2 Pt 1):233–6.
25. Farma JM, Ammori JB, Zager JS, et al. Dermatofibrosarcoma protuberans: how wide should we resect? Ann Surg Oncol 2010;17(8):2112–8.
26. Snow SN, Gordon EM, Larson PO, et al. Dermatofibrosarcoma protuberans: a report on 29 patients treated by Mohs micrographic surgery with long-term follow-up and review of the literature. Cancer 2004;101(1):28–38.
27. Stojadinovic A, Karpoff HM, Antonescu CR, et al. Dermatofibrosarcoma protuberans of the head and neck. Ann Surg Oncol 2000;7(9):696–704.
28. Wilder F, D'Angelo S, Crago AM. Soft tissue tumors of the trunk: management of local disease in the breast and chest and abdominal walls. J Surg Oncol 2015; 111(5):546–52.
29. Dagan R, Morris CG, Zlotecki RA, et al. Radiotherapy in the treatment of dermatofibrosarcoma protuberans. Am J Clin Oncol 2005;28(6):537–9.
30. Suit H, Spiro I, Mankin HJ, et al. Radiation in management of patients with dermatofibrosarcoma protuberans. J Clin Oncol 1996;14(8):2365–9.
31. Sun LM, Wang CJ, Huang CC, et al. Dermatofibrosarcoma protuberans: treatment results of 35 cases. Radiother Oncol J Eur Soc Ther Radiol Oncol 2000; 57(2):175–81.
32. Chen Y-T, Tu W-T, Lee W-R, et al. The efficacy of adjuvant radiotherapy in dermatofibrosarcoma protuberans: a systemic review and meta-analysis. J Eur Acad Dermatol Venereol 2016;30(7):1107–14.
33. Navarrete-Dechent C, Mori S, Barker CA, et al. Imatinib Treatment for Locally Advanced or Metastatic Dermatofibrosarcoma Protuberans: A Systematic Review. JAMA Dermatol 2019;155(3):361–9.
34. Kérob D, Porcher R, Vérola O, et al. Imatinib mesylate as a preoperative therapy in dermatofibrosarcoma: results of a multicenter phase II study on 25 patients. Clin Cancer Res 2010;16(12):3288–95.
35. Ugurel S, Mentzel T, Utikal J, et al. Neoadjuvant imatinib in advanced primary or locally recurrent dermatofibrosarcoma protuberans: a multicenter phase II DeCOG trial with long-term follow-up. Clin Cancer Res 2014;20(2):499–510.
36. McArthur GA. Molecular targeting of dermatofibrosarcoma protuberans: a new approach to a surgical disease. J Natl Compr Canc Netw 2007;5(5):557–62.
37. Fu Y, Kang H, Zhao H, et al. Sunitinib for patients with locally advanced or distantly metastatic dermatofibrosarcoma protuberans but resistant to imatinib. Int J Clin Exp Med 2015;8(5):8288–94.
38. Kamar FG, Kairouz VF, Sabri AN. Dermatofibrosarcoma protuberans (DFSP) successfully treated with sorafenib: case report. Clin Sarcoma Res 2013;3(1):5.
39. Delyon J, Porcher R, Battistella M, et al. A Multicenter Phase II Study of Pazopanib in Patients with Unresectable Dermatofibrosarcoma Protuberans. J Invest Dermatol 2021;141(4):761–9.e2.

The Evolving Management of Desmoid Fibromatosis

Katherine Prendergast, MD[a], Sara Kryeziu, MD[b], Aimee M. Crago, MD, PhD[c],*

KEYWORDS

- Desmoid tumor • Desmoid-type fibromatosis • Aggressive fibromatosis
- Fibromatosis • Soft tissue sarcoma

KEY POINTS

- Desmoid fibromatosis was historically managed with aggressive surgery, but the tumors have no metastatic potential and surgery can result in significant morbidity so nonoperative management is becoming standard of care in all but a small subset of cases.
- Active observation can be recommended in many patients with asymptomatic disease as a large proportion of tumors remains stable in size after an initial growth phase and a subset even regress spontaneously.
- In patients with progressive or symptomatic disease, nonoperative management may include ablative therapies or medical management with drugs such as liposomal doxorubicin or sorafenib.
- Radiation is effective in preventing disease growth, but long-term side effects related to this treatment mean it is rarely prescribed at most institutions.
- Upfront active observation may not be appropriate for intra-abdominal desmoids except in the smallest tumors as the growth of these tumors can lead to life-threatening complications; systemic therapy is generally the treatment of choice for these lesions through surgery can be considered in tumors that could be resected without injury to the central mesenteric vessels.

INTRODUCTION

Desmoid fibromatosis (also referred to as desmoid-type fibromatosis, desmoid tumor, or aggressive fibromatosis) is a rare disease affecting only about 1200 patients in the United States yearly. It is most commonly diagnosed in the second through fourth decades of life and can occur throughout the body. The tumor represents a

[a] Sarcoma Biology Laboratory, Memorial Sloan Kettering Cancer Center, 417 East 68th Street, ZRC 445, New York, NY 10065, USA; [b] Department of General Surgery, NYU Grossman School of Medicine, 550 1st Avenue, New York, NY 10016, USA; [c] Gastric and Mixed Tumor Service, Department of Surgery, Memorial Sloan Kettering Cancer Center, 1275 York Avenue, H1220, New York, NY 10065, USA
* Corresponding author.
E-mail address: cragoa@mskcc.org
Twitter: @AimeeCragoMD (A.M.C.)

Surg Clin N Am 102 (2022) 667–677
https://doi.org/10.1016/j.suc.2022.05.005
0039-6109/22/© 2022 Elsevier Inc. All rights reserved.
surgical.theclinics.com

mesenchymal lesion composed of a clonal population of cells.[1] Genomic studies have shown more than 90% of tumors are associated with a mutation in *CTNNB1*, the gene encoding the β-catenin transcription factor, or in *APC*, an upstream inhibitor of β-catenin.[2,3] Rarely, the lesion occurs in patients with germline *APC* mutation and familial adenomatous polyposis (FAP). Desmoids diagnosed in this context can also be associated with osteomas, epidermal inclusion cysts, and retinal abnormalities, a constellation referred to as Gardner's syndrome.[4,5] Under normal circumstances, β-catenin is carefully regulated by upstream, canonical Wnt signaling pathways. *APC* or *CTNNB1* mutations found in desmoid tumors prevent the degradation of β-catenin and are associated with increased levels of the nuclear form of the protein, an event which presumably leads to aberrant oncogenic transcription. Recent studies using whole-exome sequencing of desmoid tumors without *CTNNB1* or *APC* mutation show that less common events with the potential to dysregulate β-catenin and stem cell pathways are present in these lesions, supporting a central role for Wnt/β-catenin activation in desmoids.[6]

Historically, desmoids were thought to behave like soft tissue sarcoma, so were managed with aggressive surgery and cytotoxic chemotherapies. In-depth analysis of retrospective databases demonstrated, however, that the tumors have no metastatic potential and postoperatively, local recurrences were common.[7,8] For these reasons, in the absence of local symptoms, a concern predominantly in tumors found within the abdomen that can fistulize or cause obstruction or in multi-focal extremity disease known to cause debilitating limb contracture, modern management paradigms largely focus on minimizing symptoms related to locally aggressive disease.[9] Tumors that do not cause pain may, in fact, be observed after initial diagnosis since a large subset of tumors will stop growing or even regress spontaneously. When tumors do progress, become symptomatic, or grow in the abdomen, systemic therapies of significant benefit have been identified and may be prescribed to avoid the morbidity associated with major surgical resection.

PATIENT EVALUATION OVERVIEW

Patients with desmoid-type fibromatosis generally present with a painless mass as in the context of other soft tissue tumors. Most patients are in their second through fourth decades of life. The tumors can present anywhere in the body, but common scenarios include rectus sheath lesions diagnosed in the first one to 2 years after a pregnancy, extremity lesions (sometimes multifocal) in the teens and 20s, and intraabdominal masses involving the mesentery and often its central vessels. Approximately 15% are diagnosed in the postpartum period and 10% are clearly documented to be localized to the region of prior surgery or injury.[10]

Initial work-up includes cross-sectional imaging with MRI or CT to define anatomy. MRI characteristics have been associated with biologic behavior of the desmoid (see later in discussion of active observation), but CT can be particularly useful for intraabdominal lesions.[11] In this instance, surgical resection remains an important modality for the treatment and adequate assessment of tumor relationship to the mesenteric vessels is essential to determine resectability. Ability to assess vascular involvement may be limited on MRI due to motion artifacts caused by peristalsis.

While clinical history can be highly suggestive of a desmoid tumor as opposed to other subtypes of soft tissue sarcoma, biopsy is required to confirm the diagnosis. As with any soft tissue mass, these biopsies should be approached through the location of a potential surgical incision in the event that the lesion is diagnosed as a sarcoma as opposed to desmoid. Core biopsy is preferred to fine-needle aspiration as it provides adequate tissue for the assessment of tumor architecture and for use in ancillary pathologic studies. Desmoids are composed of bland fibroblasts and myofibroblasts. Cells are arranged in long fascicles and can have a dense, eosinophilic stroma. There is little atypia and few mitoses are visible (**Fig. 1**). Lesions are positive for SMA and desmoid by immunohistochemistry.[12] Approximately 80% have nuclear staining for β-catenin.[13] In cases whereby the diagnosis is equivocal, next-generation sequencing platforms can be of use in confirming the diagnosis by demonstrating canonical *CTNNB1* or *APC* mutations. *CTNNB1* mutations are generally noted to affect exon 3, most commonly seen as T41A, S45F, or S45P point mutations.[2,6,14]

At the time of desmoid diagnosis, it is important to screen patients for risk of underlying FAP. Guidelines generally suggest that a patient with a newly diagnosed desmoid should undergo colonoscopy. It is rare, however, for desmoids to be the presenting sign of FAP; development of desmoids in Gardner's patients generally occurs after surgical treatment of known polyposis. In one study, 161 patients with the new diagnosis of desmoid and no prior history of FAP were examined. Underlying FAP was found in less than 4% of patients and only in the context of multiple risk factors associated with the condition (including intraabdominal lesion, multifocal disease, family history of colorectal cancer, and age less than age 40y at the time of desmoid diagnosis). Given these findings, it may be safe to defer colonoscopy in a subset of newly diagnosed patients with desmoid with no other factors suggestive of underlying germline *APC* abnormality. The presence of *CTNNB1* mutation in a desmoid would also suggest a lesion is sporadic, not related to an inherited condition, so that with increasing use of routine genomic sequencing of tumors, colonoscopy may not be necessary for patients whose tumors screen positive for *CTNNB1* mutation as opposed to those with an abnormality in *APC* or no detectable mutation.[10]

ACTIVE OBSERVATION IN PATIENTS WITH DESMOID

Historically, patients with desmoid-type fibromatosis were treated aggressively with surgery in an attempt to cure disease or, when nonoperable, with multiple lines of systemic therapy. Side effects of these interventions could, however, be quite morbid with amputations or short bowel syndrome resulting in extreme cases. Even with aggressive procedures, rates of local recurrence were reported to be 30% to 60%. Desmoid

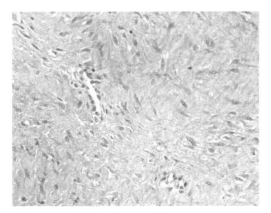

Fig. 1. Light microscopy of hematoxylin and eosin-stained desmoid section. Bland spindle cells without atypia or mitoses are observed in a densely eosinophilic background. Cells are arranged in fascicles with intermittent, thinned-walled vessels.

tumors do not metastasize and, after this fact was clearly documented, there were case reports of patients with multiply recurrent disease managed without intervention due to potential risks from further treatment.[7,8] It was also noted that even in the absence of intervention, a subset of desmoids did not grow and another subset seemed to regress spontaneously. In a large, retrospective series, 142 patients managed with active observation or medical therapy were studied. No difference in progression-free survival (PFS) was noted between groups (49.9 vs 58.6% after 5 years).[15] More recently, in the placebo-control arm of a phase III trial examining the efficacy of sorafenib in desmoid patients with recurrent or symptomatic disease or documented disease progression, an estimated 36% of patients had stable disease by RECIST criteria 2-years after enrollment and 20% of patients were noted to regress spontaneously.

Based on these data, active observation has been integrated more consistently into therapeutic paradigms. In fact, recent consensus guidelines suggest an initial period of observation would be appropriate for almost all patients with desmoid.[9] However, this should be predicated on patients being relatively asymptomatic and the tumor is located in an area whereby growth would not risk complications. Desmoids produce a high quantity of collagenous stroma that may not regress with subsequent treatment and resultant pain or limb contracture may not be reversible. Intraabdominal tumors can be life-threatening if they cause fistulization or obstruction and progressive mesenteric involvement can complicate attempts to treat life-threatening emergencies that would normally be managed with surgery.

Ideally, clinical and biologic markers that predict progression would be available to determine which patients have a disease with a high likelihood of stabilization when recommending upfront observation. Clinical characteristics such as size and site that reliably predict recurrence after desmoid resection are not universally associated with growth during observation. In addition, a poor understanding of desmoid biology has hindered attempts to develop predictive markers. In one retrospective series of 72 patients managed with active observation, size greater than 5 cm was associated with time to treatment, however, not RECIST-defined progression. MRI characteristics seemed to be the factor most closely associated with tumor growth when defined strictly by RECIST criteria. For patients with at least 90% of the tumor characterized by a hyperintense signal on T2 sequences, a factor thought to reflect a highly cellular tumor, 1-year PFS was only 55%. Tumors with lower intensity signals on T2-weighted sequences were noted to have PFS of 94% (**Fig. 2**).[11] Further prospective trials examining outcomes of active observation in patients with desmoid are being developed and plan to include radiographic and molecular correlates in an attempt to better delineate predictive markers for desmoid growth.

PHARMACOLOGIC OR MEDICAL TREATMENT OPTIONS

In patients with progressive desmoid fibromatosis, those with symptoms, or those in whom risks related to growth are significant, systemic therapies, surgery, and ablative therapies are considered. Systemic therapy is often prescribed as first-line management though the choice of intervention (eg, medical, surgical or ablative) is partially dictated by tumor location. For extremity and chest wall desmoids, systemic therapy is considered as opposed to surgery given high rates of local recurrence after resection. For intra-abdominal tumors, systemic therapy may be preferable to surgery if there is mesenteric vessel involvement or if large segments of bowel would need to be removed for complete resection of the desmoid.[16,17] Systemic therapies may be considered in patients with progressive abdominal wall lesions, but in this instance, ablative therapies are more often considered if intervention is required given the

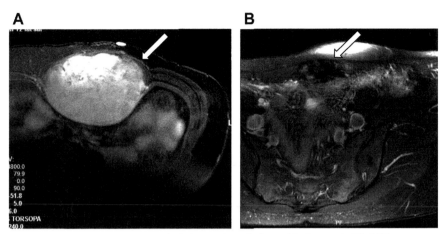

Fig. 2. Cross-sectional imaging of abdominal wall desmoids (*arrows*). T2 MRI sequences showing a lesion with (*A*) hyperintense signal that subsequently progressed and (*B*) a desmoid with low signal intensity that remained stable during active observation.

favorable anatomy and high rates of local control in what are generally small tumors (see later in discussion; **Fig. 3**).

A wide range of medical therapies has been used in the management of desmoid-type fibromatosis. Historically, patients with unresectable disease were treated with antihormonal therapy (tamoxifen), nonsteroidal antiinflammatory drugs (particularly celecoxib or sulindac), as well as cytotoxic therapies.[18] Common regimens included combinations of methotrexate and vinblastine, as well as anthracycline-, dacarbazine- and tyrosine kinase-based treatments. A study by the Pediatric Oncology Group described a phase II trial enrolling 28 patients on the vinblastine and methotrexate regimen. Clinical benefit (responses plus stable disease) was observed in 18 patients

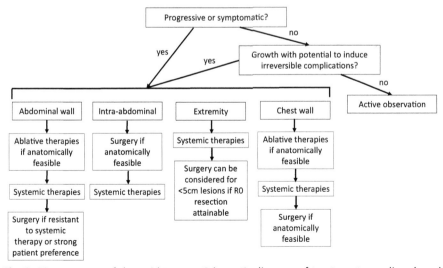

Fig. 3. Management of desmoid tumors. Schematic diagram of treatment paradigm based on the location of desmoid primary and showing example prioritization of treatment modality when intervention is required.

(64%).[19] A phase II trial examining imatinib in adult patients with desmoids showed 65% had progression arrest 6 months after the initiation of treatment (800 mg daily).[20]

The difficulty in interpreting these studies and how they should guide patient care is 2-fold. First, many of the trials and reports were performed before active observation was routinely integrated into treatment paradigms, so that patients could have had stable disease even without drug treatment. Second, the trials do not directly compare outcomes between groups of patients treated with different regimens so that relative efficacy is unclear. The question of relative efficacy was addressed in a retrospective series written by de Camargo and colleagues[21] This analysis identified 68 patients treated with 157 lines of therapy. Best responses were defined by RECIST. The highest rates of partial response were observed in patients treated with anthracycline-containing regimens (33%) and single-agent methotrexate (33%). However, clinical benefit, when defined as percent of patients with a stable or responsive disease was relatively consistent across regimens, measured at approximately 80%. For this reason, many institutions have adopted a paradigm in which lower toxicity drugs are prescribed as first-line therapy (eg, tamoxifen or celecoxib) while cytotoxic regimens are used for patients with resistant or symptomatic disease or upfront in those tumors with the potential to cause severe complications (eg, relatively large abdominal tumors).[9] Of note, anthracycline-based therapies can be given in liposomal formulations, minimizing toxicities with retained efficacy in this disease.

In addition to the above-mentioned drugs, a phase III trial examining the role of sorafenib was recently published.[22] A unique aspect of this study was that patients enrolled in the trial were symptomatic, had a recurrent disease, or had documented radiographic progression of the desmoid. Eighty-seven patients were enrolled. PFS in the sorafenib group was 81% at 2 years compared with 36% in the placebo group. Objective response rates were 33% and 30%, respectively, and the clinical benefit (rate of responsive or stable disease) for sorafenib was at least comparable to historic outcomes reported for drugs such as doxorubicin or methotrexate (98%; **Table 1**). Median time to objective response was 9.6 months, but when managed with sorafenib, patient symptoms often improved more quickly than an objective response was noted. Of note, a subset of tumors that did not respond by size showed MRI changes corresponding to increased fibrosis and decreased cellularity (less intense signal on T2 sequences). This suggests that clinical benefit may not be strictly dependent on RECIST response. Given the results of this trial, sorafenib is increasingly used as first-line therapy in patients with desmoid. Responses have been seen even with reduced dosing so that side effect profiles can generally be managed with dose reduction when necessary.

SURGICAL AND INTERVENTIONAL RADIOLOGY MANAGEMENT OF DESMOIDS

Surgery was historically used in an attempt to completely resect desmoid tumors. Rates of local recurrence have, however, been reported to be in the range of 30% to 60%. Resections were often morbid and the risk of death due to sequelae of having a desmoid tumor is limited to very select clinical scenarios. In that context, and given new options for systemic intervention, surgery currently has a relatively limited role in the management of desmoids. When performed, it should be planned with the intent to obtain microscopically negative margins. That said, retrospective series do not show a clear association between local recurrence and R1 versus R0 margins, so that an R1 margin noted on final pathologic evaluation is generally not an indication for reexcision based on our current understanding of desmoids. Nonoperative management should uniformly be considered if complete gross resection does not seem feasible based on preoperative imaging or if resection to R0 margins would be unduly morbid.

Table 1
Best response to systemic therapy in desmoids assessed by RECIST[a]

Drug Regimen	RECIST Response	RECIST Stable Disease	Clinical Benefit	PFS (Months)
Anthracycline containing[b]	37%	51%	88%	Median not reached
Methotrexate (single agent)[b]	33%	50%	83%	9.4
Vinca-containing (eg, vinorelbine)[b]	20%	60%	80%	Median not reached
Hormonal therapy[b]	23%	65%	88%	12.0
Sorafenib[c]	33%	>65%	98%	Median not reached

[a] Adapted from de Camargo et al. and Gounder et al.[21,22].
[b] Median 5.3 y follow-up, RECIST v1.
[c] Median 2.7 y follow-up, RECIST v1.1.

Selection of patients who are optimal candidates for the surgical resection of desmoids is based on several large retrospective series that describe clinical characteristics associated with a relatively low risk of recurrence after surgery.[16,17] Reproducible associations have been shown between high rates of recurrence and extremity and chest wall sites, young age and large tumor size. For example, in a study of 439 patients undergoing complete surgical resection, 5-year local recurrence-free survival (LRFS) was 69%. In patients younger than 26 years, this rate was 52% versus 81% in patients older than 65 years. Abdominal wall tumors were associated with 5-year LRFS of 90% while 40% of extremity lesions had recurred after 5 years; intraabdominal recurrences were observed in 30% of patients. LRFS was 57% for patients with tumors greater than 10 cm in diameter but 72% for those with lesions less than 5 cm in size. Each of these differences was statistically significant.[16] Results were incorporated into an externally validated, predictive nomogram which can be used to estimate the risk of recurrence in the preoperative setting. The site of mutation in CTNNB1 has been considered as an additional predictive marker for postoperative recurrence (with S45 F mutations associated with the poorest outcomes) but results of validation studies have been variable and a high correlation between mutation site and other risk factors (such as size and tumor site) make the added value of mutation status to current models unclear.[14]

In general, these data suggest that small tumors in the abdominal wall would be ideal for surgical resection given cure rates approaching 90%, but the removal of these lesions can often require major reconstruction with mesh repair. Additionally, as noted later in discussion, small abdominal wall tumors are likely to be the best candidates for ablative therapies, which may provide a less invasive first-line approach. Extremity lesions (which are often described in conjunction with similarly behaving head and neck tumors) have high rates of local recurrence and might be better managed with systemic therapies as opposed to surgery. The one instance whereby surgery can still be beneficial is for intra-abdominal desmoids that do not involve central mesenteric vessels and surgical risks do not include short bowel syndrome. A typical patient with intraabdominal disease (20–30 year age range, with a 7–10 cm tumor) would have only a 30% local recurrence risk 5 years after resection per the aforementioned nomogram, in other words, a 70% chance of cure after R0/R1 surgery.[16]

Nonoperative approaches that build on interventional radiology techniques developed in other fields are increasingly playing a role in the management of desmoid-type fibromatosis. Chemical and radiofrequency ablation, high-intensity focused ultrasound and, most recently, chemoembolization have all been studied in small series.[23-29] Currently, the best-described form of ablative therapy is cryoablation. This technique involves the image-guided insertion of a probe into the desmoid by freezing the viable cells, inducing long-term scar formation in the tumor bed. Early reports demonstrated high rates of local control with favorable toxicity profiles.[30,31] A recent retrospective series has described 22 patients with desmoid treated with cryoablation, comparing outcomes with those observed in a propensity-matched surgical cohort.[32] While local recurrence was more common after cryoablation (59% 2 years after ablation vs 71% after surgery), the ability to perform a second cryoablation procedure in the event of a small recurrence led to identical rates of long-term disease control in patients managed with cryoablation and surgery. Factors associated with the risk of recurrence included size greater than 5 cm, age 25 years or younger, and cryoablation for recurrent disease. All patients with 2 or more of these risk factors were observed to have a local recurrence 2.5 years after the procedure, while none of the patients with no risk factors or only one risk factor recurred. These data confirm that cryoablation is ideal for small, primary tumors in regions such as the chest or abdominal wall whereby there is little risk of injury to adjacent neurovascular structures and underlying organs can be pushed away from the treatment site using hydrodissection.

RADIATION THERAPY FOR DESMOIDS

Radiation in the adjuvant setting is highly controversial and not generally pursued at major academic centers. Its association with improved outcomes is not reproducible in large, retrospective series. That said, desmoid tumors do seem to be radiosensitive. In a retrospective analysis of patients with desmoid treated at MD Anderson Cancer Center, 41 patients were treated with definitive radiation (median dose 56 Gy) and 74 were treated with combined surgery and radiation (median dose 50 Gy).[33] The 5-year LRFS rates were 75% and did not differ significantly between the 2 cohorts. Based on these data, definitive radiation is considered an option for patients with progressive desmoid fibromatosis.

Radiation is used in a highly selective manner at most major academic centers given the risk of significant side effects in a young patient population. Joint fibrosis and bone fracture can be difficult to manage and result in an irreversible compromise on the quality of life. Perhaps more significantly, radiation-associated sarcomas have been noted to develop in a subset of patients during long-term follow-up. These tumors can be difficult to resect given not only innate anatomic limitations but also due to related desmoplastic changes in the surgical field that result from the initial desmoid tumor as well as surrounding radiation-associated fibrosis.

NEW DEVELOPMENTS

Current research seeking to refine the therapeutic paradigms for patients with desmoid is focused on developing novel therapeutics, identifying predictive markers for tumor response to therapy and defining subsets of tumors most likely to progress during periods of active observation. In addition to sorafenib, a recent phase II clinical trial has shown the efficacy of gamma-secretase inhibitors (nirogacestat) and ongoing studies are examining toxicities in patients with desmoid treated with direct inhibitors of beta-catenin (tegavivint).[34,35] It is unclear why treatment with either sorafenib or gamma-secretase inhibitors would be effective in desmoids, making it difficult to predict which tumors may be most responsive to the drugs. Ongoing translational studies are examining these questions while also attempting to better define the subset of tumors most at risk of progressing during periods of active observation.

SUMMARY

The management of desmoid fibromatosis has evolved rapidly over the last decade. While previously treated with aggressive surgery, current paradigms suggest most tumors can be managed with an initial period of active observation as the tumors do not metastasize and may regress spontaneously. In cases whereby tumors progress, are symptomatic, or whereby growth would have the potential to cause significant complications, nonoperative management strategies such as sorafenib or cryoablation can be used to minimize treatment morbidity. With continued research examining the molecular underpinnings of β-catenin induced oncogenesis in desmoids, a better understanding of which patients respond best to which therapies can be expected with even more precise tailoring of therapy developed for patients in the future.

CLINICS CARE POINTS

- Active observation is considered first-line therapy for most desmoids. Exceptions include tumors that are symptomatic or that have the potential to cause significant symptoms with growth (eg, intraabdominal lesions that may obstruct or fistulize).

- Surgery remains an option for intraabdominal lesions that do not involve the central mesentery and could be resected without a significant portion of the bowel.

- Nonoperative interventions include medical therapies such as liposomal doxorubicin or sorafenib which are ideal for patients with unresectable disease or tumors that are associated with a high risk of local recurrence such as those in the extremity.

- Cryoablation is effective in controlling small tumors in anatomically favorable locations such as the abdominal and chest walls; chemoembolization and high-intensity focused ultrasound are used to treat selected patients at some institutions.

- While effective, radiation can cause long-term side effects and radiation-associated sarcomas. These risks should be carefully weighed before prescribing radiation for patients with desmoid, who tend to be young.

FUNDING STATEMENT

This work was funded in part by the following NIH/NCI grants 5T32CA009501(K. Prendergast), 5R37CA241856(A. M. Crago), the MSKCC SPORE in Soft Tissue Sarcoma (5P50CA217694), and the MSKCC Cancer Center grant (5P30CA008748).

DISCLOSURE

K. Prendergast – nothing to disclose S. Kryeziu – nothing to disclose A.M. Crago – advisory board, Springworks Therapeutics.

REFERENCES

1. Alman BA, Pajerski ME, Diaz-Cano S, et al. Aggressive fibromatosis (desmoid tumor) is a monoclonal disorder. Diagn Mol Pathol 1997;6:98–101.
2. Alman BA, Li C, Pajerski ME, et al. Increased beta-catenin protein and somatic APC mutations in sporadic aggressive fibromatoses (desmoid tumors). Am J Pathol 1997;151:329–34.
3. Couture J, Mitri A, Lagace R, et al. A germline mutation at the extreme 3' end of the APC gene results in a severe desmoid phenotype and is associated with over-expression of beta-catenin in the desmoid tumor. Clin Genet 2000;57:205–12.

4. Gardner EJ, Richards RC. Multiple cutaneous and subcutaneous lesions occurring simultaneously with hereditary polyposis and osteomatosis. Am J Hum Genet 1953;5:139–47.
5. Nishisho I, Nakamura Y, Miyoshi Y, et al. Mutations of chromosome 5q21 genes in FAP and colorectal cancer patients. Science 1991;253:665–9.
6. Crago AM, Chmielecki J, Rosenberg M, et al. Near universal detection of alterations in CTNNB1 and Wnt pathway regulators in desmoid-type fibromatosis by whole-exome sequencing and genomic analysis. Genes Chromosomes Cancer 2015;54:606–15.
7. Lewis JJ, Boland PJ, Leung DH, et al. The enigma of desmoid tumors. Ann Surg 1999;229:866–72 [discussion: 872–873].
8. Merchant NB, Lewis JJ, Woodruff JM, et al. Extremity and trunk desmoid tumors: a multifactorial analysis of outcome. Cancer 1999;86:2045–52.
9. Desmoid Tumor Working G. The management of desmoid tumours: a joint global consensus-based guideline approach for adult and paediatric patients. Eur J Cancer 2020;127:96–107.
10. van Houdt WJ, Wei IH, Kuk D, et al. Yield of colonoscopy in identification of newly diagnosed desmoid-type fibromatosis with underlying familial adenomatous polyposis. Ann Surg Oncol 2019;26:765–71.
11. Cassidy MR, Lefkowitz RA, Long N, et al. Association of MRI T2 signal intensity with desmoid tumor progression during active observation: a retrospective cohort study. Ann Surg 2018;271(4):748–55.
12. Fritchie KJ, Crago AM, van de Rijn M. Desmoid fibromatosis. In: Board TWCoTE, editor. WHO Classification of tumours: soft tissue and bone tumours. Lyon, France: International Agency for Research on Cancer; 2020. p. 93–5.
13. Ng TL, Gown AM, Barry TS, et al. Nuclear beta-catenin in mesenchymal tumors. Mod Pathol 2005;18:68–74.
14. Lazar AJ, Tuvin D, Hajibashi S, et al. Specific mutations in the beta-catenin gene (CTNNB1) correlate with local recurrence in sporadic desmoid tumors. Am J Pathol 2008;173:1518–27.
15. Fiore M, Rimareix F, Mariani L, et al. Desmoid-type fibromatosis: a front-line conservative approach to select patients for surgical treatment. Ann Surg Oncol 2009;16:2587–93.
16. Crago AM, Denton B, Salas S, et al. A prognostic nomogram for prediction of recurrence in desmoid fibromatosis. Ann Surg 2013;258:347–53.
17. Salas S, Dufresne A, Bui B, et al. Prognostic factors influencing progression-free survival determined from a series of sporadic desmoid tumors: a wait-and-see policy according to tumor presentation. J Clin Oncol 2011;29:3553–8.
18. Hansmann A, Adolph C, Vogel T, et al. High-dose tamoxifen and sulindac as first-line treatment for desmoid tumors. Cancer 2004;100:612–20.
19. Skapek SX, Ferguson WS, Granowetter L, et al. Vinblastine and methotrexate for desmoid fibromatosis in children: results of a Pediatric Oncology Group Phase II Trial. J Clin Oncol 2007;25:501–6.
20. Kasper B, Gruenwald V, Reichardt P, et al. Imatinib induces sustained progression arrest in RECIST progressive desmoid tumours: Final results of a phase II study of the German Interdisciplinary Sarcoma Group (GISG). Eur J Cancer 2017;76:60–7.
21. de Camargo VP, Keohan ML, D'Adamo DR, et al. Clinical outcomes of systemic therapy for patients with deep fibromatosis (desmoid tumor). Cancer 2010;116:2258–65.

22. Gounder MM, Mahoney MR, Van Tine BA, et al. Sorafenib for Advanced and Refractory Desmoid Tumors. N Engl J Med 2018;379:2417–28.
23. Clark TW. Percutaneous chemical ablation of desmoid tumors. J Vasc Interv Radiol 2003;14:629–34.
24. Tsz-Kan T, Man-Kwong C, Shu Shang-Jen J, et al. Radiofrequency ablation of recurrent fibromatosis. J Vasc Interv Radiol 2007;18:147–50.
25. Ilaslan H, Schils J, Joyce M, et al. Radiofrequency ablation: another treatment option for local control of desmoid tumors. Skeletal Radiol 2010;39:169–73.
26. Avedian RS, Bitton R, Gold G, et al. Is MR-guided high-intensity focused ultrasound a feasible treatment modality for desmoid tumors? Clin Orthop Relat Res 2016;474:697–704.
27. Anastas JN, Kulikauskas RM, Tamir T, et al. WNT5A enhances resistance of melanoma cells to targeted BRAF inhibitors. J Clin Invest 2014;124:2877–90.
28. Wang Y, Wang W, Tang J. Ultrasound-guided high intensity focused ultrasound treatment for extra-abdominal desmoid tumours: preliminary results. Int J Hyperthermia 2011;27:648–53.
29. Elnekave E, Atar E, Amar S, et al. Doxorubicin-eluting intra-arterial therapy for pediatric extra-abdominal desmoid fibromatoses: a promising approach for a perplexing disease. J Vasc Interv Radiol 2018;29:1376–82.
30. Havez M, Lippa N, Al-Ammari S, et al. Percutaneous image-guided cryoablation in inoperable extra-abdominal desmoid tumors: a study of tolerability and efficacy. Cardiovasc Intervent Radiol 2014;37(6):1500–6.
31. Kujak JL, Liu PT, Johnson GB, et al. Early experience with percutaneous cryoablation of extra-abdominal desmoid tumors. Skeletal Radiol 2010;39:175–82.
32. Mandel JE, Kim D, Yarmohammadi H, et al. Percutaneous Cryoablation Provides Disease Control for Extra-Abdominal Desmoid-Type Fibromatosis Comparable with Surgical Resection. Ann Surg Oncol 2022;29:640–8.
33. Guadagnolo BA, Zagars GK, Ballo MT. Long-term outcomes for desmoid tumors treated with radiation therapy. Int J Radiat Oncol Biol Phys 2008;71:441–7.
34. Kummar S, O'Sullivan Coyne G, Do KT, et al. Clinical activity of the gamma-secretase inhibitor PF-03084014 in adults with desmoid tumors (aggressive fibromatosis). J Clin Oncol 2017;35:1561–9.
35. Villalobos VM, Hall F, Jimeno A, et al. Long-Term Follow-Up of Desmoid Fibromatosis Treated with PF-03084014, an Oral Gamma Secretase Inhibitor. Ann Surg Oncol 2018;25:768–75.

Benign Neurogenic Tumors

Jeffrey M. Farma, MD*, Andrea S. Porpiglia, MD, Elaine T. Vo, MD

KEYWORDS

- Benign neurogenic tumors • Pheochromocytoma • Paraganglioma • Schwannoma
- Neurofibroma

KEY POINTS

- Neurogenic tumors are most commonly found in the posterior mediastinum and the retroperitoneum.
- Surgeons should have pheochromocytomas and paragangliomas as a differential for adrenal masses and para-aortic masses.
- The main modality of treatment for neurogenic tumors is surgical resection.

INTRODUCTION

Neurogenic tumors arise from cells that make up the nervous system. These tumors account for approximately 12% of all benign and 8% of all malignant soft tissue neoplasms.[1] The location is related to distribution of the peripheral nervous system, which is made up of the autonomic nervous system (sympathetic and parasympathetic system) and somatic nervous system. In the abdomen, they are most commonly located in the retroperitoneum, specifically the paraspinal/para-aortic region, and adrenal glands.[2]

Neurogenic tumors are classified based on their origin cells: ganglion cells (ganglioneuroma, ganglioneuroblastoma, neuroblastoma), paraganglion cells (pheochromocytomas, paragangliomas), and nerve sheath cells (neurilemmomas/schwannomas, neurofibromas, neurofibromatosis [NF]).[2] The incidence of neurogenic tumors is not reported; however, it is known that primary intrathoracic neurogenic tumors account for 95% of all posterior mediastinal tumors.[3] Abdominal neurogenic tumors generally follow the distribution of the sympathetic ganglia along the paraspinal areas and can arise from the adrenal medulla or the organ of Zuckerkandl.[2] Although benign, neurogenic tumors can grow and cause compression of surrounding structures depending on their location, and can even cause varying degrees of neurologic symptoms including pain, paresthesia, and weakness. Although rare, there is also the potential for malignant transformation.[2,4,5]

Fox Chase Cancer Center, 333 Cottman Avenue, Philadelphia, PA 19111, USA
* Corresponding author.
E-mail address: Jeffrey.Farma@fccc.edu

Surg Clin N Am 102 (2022) 679–693
https://doi.org/10.1016/j.suc.2022.04.007
0039-6109/22/© 2022 Elsevier Inc. All rights reserved.

surgical.theclinics.com

PATIENT EVALUATION

Benign neurogenic tumors are usually discovered as an incidental finding on cross-sectional imaging. A thorough history and physical examination should focus on neurologic compressive symptoms depending on the location of the tumor such as pain, paresthesia, or weakness. The presence of pain, significant neurologic deficits, weight loss, or a heterogeneous mass is more concerning for a malignant process. Examination for the presence of cutaneous neurofibromas should be noted. Neurogenic tumors can present as a component of genetic syndromes. Therefore, it is important to consider a family history of or previously undiagnosed genetic disorders such as NF-1 and NF-2.

Initial evaluation with ultrasonography is reasonable, primarily for cutaneous lesions. Definitive imaging with cross-sectional imaging with either computed tomography (CT) with intravenous contrast or MRI with and without contrast is recommended for preoperative planning.[6] Given the difficulty of evaluating the difference between benign and malignant tumors on imaging, biopsy is frequently recommended. In tumors located close to the spinal column, it is important to evaluate for intraspinal extension of the tumor. In these circumstances, MRI is the modality of choice to assess for intraforaminal involvement of the tumor.[3] If intraforaminal involvement is present, consultation with orthopedic or neurosurgery is appropriate.

If clinically indicated (progressive enlargement, associated pain, or other symptoms), surgical excision of a benign neurogenic tumor with grossly negative margins is an appropriate treatment. If possible, the capsule can be incised in a longitudinal fashion and the parent nerve fascicle in which the tumor arises can be identified/preserved. However, if the capsule is densely adherent, it is acceptable to perform a subtotal resection, leaving residual disease to preserve nerves and prevent major morbidity.[5]

CLASSIFICATION OF NEUROGENIC TUMORS
Ganglion Cells: Neuroblastomas, Ganglioneuroblastomas, and Ganglioneuromas

Neurogenic tumors of ganglion cell origin are derived from neural crest cells. Based on the International Neuroblastoma Pathology Classification (1999) by the International Neuroblastoma Pathology Committee, there are 4 categories of peripheral neuroblastic tumors: neuroblastoma, ganglioneuroblastoma, ganglioneuroblastoma nodular, and ganglioneuroma.[7] Neuroblastomas and ganglioneuroblastomas often occur in infants and children. Ganglioneuromas are usually present in adolescents and young adults.[8]

Neuroblastomas and ganglioneuroblastomas are considered malignant diseases. There are approximately 500 to 525 new cases of neuroblastomas each year in the United States, and it is the third most common pediatric malignancy. The most common sites of origin of neuroblastomas and ganglioneuroblastomas are the adrenal medulla (35% of cases), extra-adrenal retroperitoneum (30%–35%), and posterior mediastinum (20%). Less common sites include the neck (1%–5% of cases) and pelvis (2%–3%).[9] Neuroblastomas have the most immature, undifferentiated cells and are generally considered malignant. Neuroblastomas tend to be more aggressive and seen in younger patients. The median age at diagnosis is 17 months.[9] Ganglioneuroblastomas have intermediate malignant potential and contain both mature gangliocytes and immature neuroblasts. As this article focuses on benign neurogenic tumors, the staging and treatment of neuroblastoma and ganglioneuroblastoma are not discussed.

Ganglioneuromas are considered benign and composed of gangliocytes and mature stroma.[8,10] Compared with neuroblastoma and ganglioneuroblastoma, these are often seen in older children with reported means ranging from the first to the fifth decades of life.[11] Ganglioneuroblastoma are typically found in children older than 10 years.[12] Fliedner and colleagues[11] performed a systematic review on ganglioneuromas, and the mean age of diagnosis was 31.2 years. Ganglioneuromas are often sporadic; however, some are associated with multiple endocrinologic neoplasia type II or NF-2.[10] Ganglioneuromas were estimated to account for 4% of adrenal incidentalomas with a prevalence of approximately 2%.[11,13] Ganglioneuromas can arise on their own or from neuroblastomas and ganglioneuroblastomas. In some cases, they have been found after radiation. The most common locations are the posterior mediastinum (40%) and the retroperitoneum (30%–50%). Adrenal glands account for 20% to 25% of reported cases, and cervical region, for around 8% to 9%.[8] These tumors have vague symptoms and often present as an incidental finding.[11] In up to 39% to 57% of ganglioneuromas, there have been reports of an association with elevated blood and urine levels of homovanillic acid and/or vanillylmandelic acid (VMA), and also potential tumor uptake of the norepinephrine analogue, metaiodobenzylguanidine (MIBG).[8,11] However, this is more common with neuroblastomas or ganglioneuroblastomas, occurring in 90% to 95% of patients.[8]

On imaging, it is difficult to differentiate between neuroblastomas, ganglioneuroblastomas, and ganglioneuromas. On ultrasonography, ganglioneuromas usually are represented as a homogeneous, hypoechoic mass with well-defined borders. On CT, calcifications may be seen in 42% to 60% of ganglioneuromas. On MRI, ganglioneuromas demonstrate low intensity on T1-weighted imaging and heterogeneous high signal on T2-weighted images (**Fig. 1**). MRI is the preferred modality to evaluate for intraspinal extension.[8] Surgical resection is the mainstay of treatment with a very low risk for future recurrence.[10] Complete resection can be achieved in up to 89% of patients.[11] There are conflicting recommendations in the literature on long-term follow-up (see **Fig. 1**; **Fig. 2**).

Paraganglion Cells: Pheochromocytomas and Paragangliomas

Pheochromocytomas and paragangliomas are very rare tumors. However, the clinician must include these entities on their differential diagnosis preoperatively due to potential significant blood pressure risks with anesthesia. Pheochromocytomas are catecholamine-secreting tumors that arise from chromaffin cells,[14] generally arising

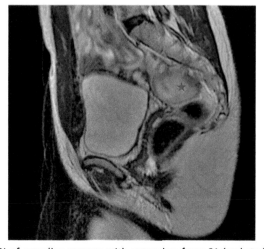

Fig. 1. Sagittal MRI of ganglioneuroma with extension from S1 (*red star*).

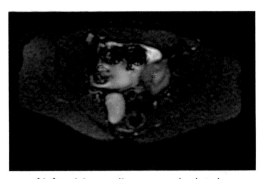

Fig. 2. MRI axial image of left pelvic ganglioneuroma (*red star*).

from the adrenal glands. Paragangliomas are rare neuroendocrine tumors that are derived from extra-adrenal chromaffin cells in sympathoadrenal and parasympathetic paraganglia.[15–18] These tumors generally originate in carotid and aortic bodies, the organ of Zuckerlandl, and other unnamed paraganglia.[19] Paragangliomas that arise in the head and neck region are typically symptomatic tumors found at the carotid bifurcation, followed by the ganglion nodosum.[19,20] However, paragangliomas of the retroperitoneum most commonly are para-aortic in location.[19] Paragangliomas in general do not produce catecholamines when compared with pheochromocytomas, which produce any combination of epinephrine, norepinephrine, and dopamine.[15]

The incidence of pheochromocytoma and paraganglioma is estimated to be 0.66 cases per 100,000 people per year.[21] Peak age is in the third to fifth decades of life.[22] Approximately 70% are sporadic and 30% are associated with a hereditary syndrome.[23] However, more recent studies demonstrate higher rates of germline mutations, which can be detected in 47% to 54.4% of patients.[22,24] The most common mutation associated with paragangliomas and pheochromocytoma is SDHB mutation, followed by SDHD, NF1, VHL, RET, SDHC, and TMEM127 mutations.[22,23] SDHD mutations are more likely to be multifocal and are usually seen in the head and neck region with low malignant potential.[25] In contrast, SDHB mutations are associated with a 25% to 50% risk of malignancy.[25] Patients with a mutation are more likely to be diagnosed at a younger age.[22] Carney triad is 3 types of neoplasms: gastric gastrointestinal stromal tumor, pulmonary chondromas, and extra-adrenal paragangliomas. There is also an increased risk of pheochromocytoma, esophageal leiomyoma, and adrenocortical adenomas. In contrast, Carney-Stratakis syndrome is a hereditary syndrome associated with germline mutations in the mitochondrial tumor suppressor gene. It cannot be highlighted enough that genetic testing should be performed on all patients with pheochromocytomas or paragangliomas.

Malignant disease is present in about 5% to 10% of adrenal pheochromocytomas and about 15% to 42% of paragangliomas.[26–29] A malignant diagnosis is defined by metastatic disease to lymph nodes, bones, liver, lung, and/or brain.[23] Those with genetic mutations have synchronous metastatic disease in approximately 11% of pheochromocytoma cases and in 31% of patients with paragangliomas.[23] There are no clear prognostic factors to determine recurrence or mortality. Factors associated with rapid disease progression and mortality in a multivariate analysis by Hamidi and colleagues[23] included older age at diagnosis, larger tumors, and synchronous metastases. The 5-year overall survival for malignant pheochromocytoma and paragangliomas ranges from 58% to 85.4%.[23,30,31]

Pheochromocytoma of the adrenal gland scaled score (PASS) was developed to formulate a guide to determine between benign and malignant pheochromocytomas.[14] PASS score includes necrosis (2 points), large nests or diffuse growth (2 points), high cellularity (2 points), tumor cell spindling (2 points), greater than 3 mitoses per 10 high-power field (HPF) (2 points), atypical mitotic figures (2 points), cellular monotony (2 points), extension into adipose tissue (2 points), vascular invasion (1 point), capsular invasion (1 point), nuclear pleomorphism (1 point), and nuclear hyperchromasia (1 point).[14] A PASS score less than 4 correctly identified benign tumors, and conversely, a PASS score greater than 4 predicted malignant behavior.[14] In the study by Thompson[14] to develop PASS, the 5-year disease free survival was 36%. The downside to using PASS is it does not account for extra-adrenal paragangliomas. The Grading System for Adrenal Pheochromocytoma and Paraganglioma (GAPP) is another scoring system using Ki-67 and catecholamine profile.[25,32] Limitations of these scores include that molecular data are not included in either PASS or GAPP.[25] Furthermore, GAPP has not been clinically validated.[25]

The clinical presentation of pheochromocytomas includes hypertension, headache, palpitations, chest pain, a feeling of panic or anxiety, flushing, diarrhea, nausea, or fever.[26,27,29,33] Frequently, patients have had a longstanding history of hypertension and are on multiple antihypertensive medications. Hypertension that is sustained or paroxysmal is often seen with pheochromocytomas.[33] Patients with dopamine-secreting tumors can be normotensive or even have hypotension.[26,34] Cardiovascular complications from pheochromocytomas include hypertensive crises, shock, arrhythmias, cardiomyopathy, and very rarely either sudden death or pheochromocytoma multisystem crisis.[26,35] For those patients with nonfunctioning tumors, presentation usually includes compressive symptoms from larger disease.[23] Furthermore, head and neck paragangliomas can present with pulsatile tinnitus or hearing loss.[20]

Diagnostic laboratory studies include plasma or urinary metanephrines, catecholamines, and/or VMA.[28] False-positives could be a result of certain medications; a list of these medications can be found in **Table 1**.[36] These medications should be held for at least 2 weeks before biochemical workup.[36] If metanephrine levels are not diagnostic, then the next step would be to perform a clonidine suppression test.[28,37] Clonidine normally suppresses the sympathetic nervous system; however, in patients with pheochromocytomas, plasma norepinephrine/normetanephrine will not be suppressed.[37] Normal suppression is considered if plasma normetanephrine/norepinephrine is suppressed more than 40% from baseline values.[15,28]

Further workup should include tumor localization either with an MRI or CT scan. MRI with and without contrast is preferred for extra-adrenal tumors, specifically in the skull base or neck, children, or tumors in pregnancy.[15,26] ^{123}I-MIBG scintigraphy can be

Table 1	
List of medications resulting in a false-positive for plasma metanephrines	
Tricyclic Antidepressants	Alpha-Methyldopa
Acetaminophen	Buspirone
Phenoxybenzamine	Monoamine inhibitors
Labetalol	Cocaine
Sotalol	Sulfasalazine
Sympathomimetics	Levodopa

Ref for table.[38,46]

used for patients with metastatic disease, those at increased risk for metastases (large tumor size, extra-adrenal, multifocal disease), or if the patient has recurrent disease.[15] However, several studies have demonstrated improved sensitivity for PET with flu-deoxyglucose F 18 (^{18}F-FDG PET)/CT compared with ^{123}I-MIBG in patients with met-astatic disease and, per the Endocrine Society, 18F-FDG PET/CT is the preferred modality.[15] Newer modalities for localization, include ^{68}Ga-DOTATATE PET/CT. Archier and colleagues[38] performed a prospective study in which patients were eval-uated by ^{18}F-FDOPA PET/CT; CT scan of the chest, abdomen, and pelvis; head and neck MRI (if indicated); and ^{68}Ga-DOTATATE PET/CT. The investigators found that in head and neck paragangliomas, ^{68}Ga-DOTATATE PET/CT had a higher rate of sensi-tivity than ^{18}F-FDOPA PET/CT as well as a higher rate of sensitivity for pheochromo-cytomas. Lesion-based sensitivities were 93% for ^{68}Ga-DOTATATE PET/CT and 89% for ^{18}F-FDOPA PET/CT[38] (**Figs. 3–6**).

Treatment
The first step for any patient with a functional pheochromocytoma should be to control hypertension with the initiation of an alpha-adrenergic receptor blockade such as phe-noxybenzamine.[15,29,36] The starting dose of phenoxybenzamine is 10 mg by mouth twice a day, and this can be titrated up every 2 to 3 days by 10 to 20 mg up to 30 mg 3 times a day.[26,36] Beta-blockade should only be used after patient is normo-tensive on alpha-adrenergic blockade and if the patient still has persistent tachy-cardia.[29] If beta-blockade is started before alpha-blockade, this can result in a hypertensive crisis or cardiopulmonary collapse.[26,36,39] In addition, patients with func-tioning tumors can be hypovolemic. Therefore, to increase blood volume, patients should increase fluid intake and start a high-sodium diet (5000 mg/d).[36,39] The high-sodium diet should be initiated 3 days before start of alpha-blockade.[39] The criteria to ensure appropriate preoperative preparation are listed in **Box 1**.

Surgical resection is the mainstay of treatment. Pheochromocytomas will require an adrenalectomy; if there is any evidence of local invasion then en bloc resection of adja-cent organs should be performed. Several studies have demonstrated that minimally invasive surgery is safe. Kercher and colleagues[40] prospectively studied 81 patients with pheochromocytomas or paragangliomas from 1995 to 2004 treated with laparo-scopic adrenalectomy. The complication rate was 7.5% with no perioperative blood transfusion, the conclusion being that laparoscopic adrenalectomy is safe.[40] A recent meta-analysis from Fu and colleagues[41] included 14 studies comparing laparoscopic

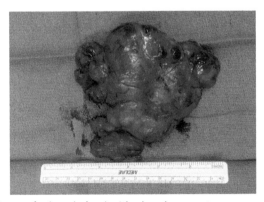

Fig. 3. Gross specimen of adrenal gland with pheochromocytoma.

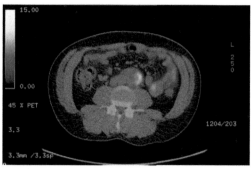

Fig. 4. ^{68}Ga-DOTATATE PET/CT demonstrating metabolically active left para-aortic heterogeneous mass consistent with known paraganglioma.

versus open resection, demonstrating more stable hemodynamics, less intraoperative blood loss, and lower overall complication rates with laparoscopic resection. Limitations of this study included inherent selection bias, and most studies reviewed were small single-institution series that only included unilateral localized adrenal pheochromocytoma.[41] Owing to the rarity of this disease, there are limited data on the use of robotic surgery for pheochromocytomas/paragangliomas. There is one prospective study from Aliyev and colleagues[42] at Cleveland Clinic that also included 25 patients who underwent robotic-assisted adrenalectomy. The tumors were less than 6 cm, and conversion rates to open were similar. The morbidity rates were 10% for the laparoscopic group and 0% for the robotic group ($P = .041$). Mortality was 2.5% for the laparoscopic group and 0% for the robotic group. This study concluded that robotic adrenalectomy is safe in patients with pheochromocytoma.[42] A limitation included that this was a prospective database but reviewed retrospectively and that it was not a randomized trial.

Morbidity after surgery can be as high as 33%.[43] Postoperatively patients should be monitored in the intensive care unit due to the risk of hypotension and hypoglycemia.[26] Patients should be assessed annually with plasma-free metanephrines or 24-h urine metanephrines.[25] There are mixed recommendations for the use of chromogranin-A as a tumor marker.

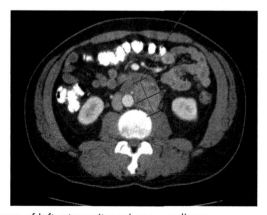

Fig. 5. Axial CT image of left retroperitoneal paraganglioma.

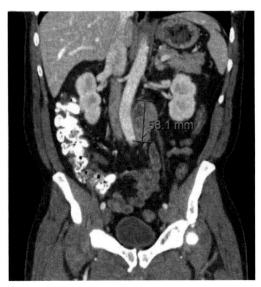

Fig. 6. Coronal CT image of left retroperitoneal paraganglioma causing deviation of aorta to the right.

Metastatic disease

About 10% to 35% of pheochromocytomas/paragangliomas are unresectable or metastatic at the time of diagnosis.[44] In this situation, one treatment option is high-specific-activity ^{131}I-MIBG.[44] A multicenter phase 2 trial evaluating the efficacy of ^{131}I-MIBG in 74 patients found that 22% had persistent antitumor effects and the 5-year overall survival for the cohort was 36%. The most common serious adverse events included hematologic toxicities (19%), pulmonary embolism (3%), and myelodysplastic syndrome (4%).[44]

Additional therapeutic options include chemotherapy. MD Anderson published a single-institution experience of chemotherapy in 52 patients with metastatic pheochromocytomas and paragangliomas, excluding head and neck paragangliomas. There were 9 patients with SDHB mutation; none of these patients responded to chemotherapy. Chemotherapy regimens varied and included platinum-based agents, cyclophosphamide, hydroxydaunorubicin, vincristine, and prednisone; temozolomide; etoposide; imatinib; ifosfamide; and thalidomide. Only 33% of patients responded to front-line chemotherapy. All patients who did have a response had

---

Box 1
Criteria for appropriate preoperative preparation

BP less than 160/90 mm Hg for at least 24 hours

Orthostatic hypotension, BP should not drop less than 80/45 mm Hg upright

No S-T segment changes and T wave inversion on ECG for 1 week

No more than one ventricular extrasystole every 5 minutes

Abbreviations: BP, blood pressure; ECG, electrocardiography.

Ref for table.[26]

regimens that included cyclophosphamide and dacarbazine. Overall survival in this cohort was 51% at 5 –years, and synchronous disease portended a worse prognosis.[45]

Nerve Sheath Cells: Neurofibromas, Neurofibromatosis, and Schwannomas

Benign peripheral nerve tumors include schwannomas (also known as neurilemmomas), neurofibromas, and NF. These tumors represent about 10% to 12% of all benign soft tissue neoplasms.[1,5] Malignant peripheral nerve sheath tumors (MPNST) represent 5% to 10% of soft tissue sarcomas and can arise from neurofibromas and, rarely, schwannomas.[5]

Schwann cells are derived from neural crest cells, and they function to myelinate peripheral nerves and serve as glial cells for the peripheral nervous system.[47] Each Schwann cell makes up a single myelin sheath on a peripheral axon. Schwannomas arise from Schwann cells and are the most common type of peripheral nerve sheath tumor, making up 5% of all benign soft tissue neoplasms.[6] Schwannomas can occur in the head and neck region as vestibular schwannomas, in the gastrointestinal tract, and even the biliary tract; they commonly occur in patients during the second and third decade of life with men and women being equally affected.[5] Schwannomas are generally solitary lesions, well circumscribed, encapsulated, and freely mobile on palpation except at the point of nerve attachment.[48] Pain and neurologic symptoms are uncommon because schwannomas do not invade the nerve. Schwannomas can produce symptoms due to compression of the nerve.[47] In a small percentage of patients with multiple schwannomas, plexiform growth and an association with NF-1 have been seen, although this is rare.[49]

The classic histologic finding for schwannomas is identification of Antoni A and Antoni B regions. Antoni A regions appear more organized and are made up of cellular spindle cells arranged in short bundles or interlacing fascicles.[5] Antoni B regions are less cellular, less organized, and contain more myxoid and loosely arranged tissue.[5] Schwann cells also characteristically stain for S-100 on immunohistochemical analysis.[5,47] Different histologic variations include ancient schwannoma, cellular schwannoma, and melanotic schwannoma.[50] Although generally benign, there is rare chance (10%) of developing into a malignant schwannoma.[6,48]

Neurofibromas are more diffuse and can involve single or multiple nerve fascicles. Often, the nerve of origin is nonfunctional at presentation because neurofibromas are more likely to infiltrate the nerve than schwannomas.[47] Neurofibromas can be classified into 3 categories: solitary, diffuse, and plexiform.[5] On histologic examination, the presence of axons within the tumor distinguishes it from schwannomas. In addition, neurofibromas do not contain Antoni A or Antoni B regions and often lack a capsule.[50] Neurofibromas can stain positive for S-100.[5] Solitary neurofibromas present as small polypoid masses. Diffuse neurofibromas have a more plaquelike appearance. Plexiform neurofibromas are large, complex, with a "bag of worms" appearance, and generally occur near large spinal roots.[5] Solitary neurofibromas rarely progress to MPNST; however, in the diffuse type, progression has been associated with multiple local recurrences.[5]

NF is a distinct and well-described group of autosomal dominant genetic syndromes caused by mutations in *neurofibromin* (NF-1) or *NF2 suppressor gene* (NF-2). NF can predispose to benign and malignant neurogenic tumors. There are 3 types of NF: NF-1, NF-2, and schwannomatosis. Schwannomatosis is a condition found in patients prone to nonvestibular schwannomas.[51]

NF-1 is the most common of the 3 conditions (1 in 3000–4000 people worldwide) and accounts for 96% of all NF syndromes.[51] NF-1 is also known as von

> **Box 2**
> **Diagnostic criteria for neurofibromatosis type 1**
>
> A. If 2 or more are present in individuals without a parent diagnosed with NF-1
> • At least 6 café-au-lait macules (>5 mm diameter in prepubertal individuals and > 15 mm in postpubertal individuals)
> • Freckling in axillary or inguinal regions[a]
> • Optic glioma
> • At least 2 Lisch nodules identified by slit lamp examination or 2 or more choroidal abnormalities
> • At least 2 neurofibromas of any type, or one plexiform neurofibroma
> • A distinctive osseous lesion such as sphenoid dysplasia, anterolateral bowing of the tibia, or pseudoarthrosis of a long bone
> • A heterozygous pathogenic NF-1 variant with a variant allele fraction of 50% in apparently normal tissue such as white blood cells
>
> B. A child of a parent who meets diagnostic criteria as specified previously and who also has 1 or more of the aforementioned criteria
>
> [a]If only café-au-lait macules and freckling are present, the diagnosis is most likely NF-1; however, consider Legius syndrome. At least 1 of the 2 pigmentary findings (café-au-lait macules or freckling) should be bilateral.
>
> Ref for table.[51]

Recklinghausen disease. NF-1 has a strong association with MPSNT, occurring in 2% to 10% of patients with NF-1. NF-1 is a genetic disorder that causes multiple tumors of nerve tissues including brain, spinal cord, and peripheral nerves. NF-1 is characterized by neurofibromas that induce skin changes and bone deformation. The characteristic

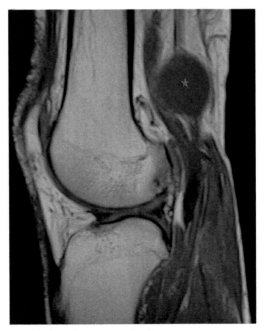

Fig. 7. MRI of lower extremity schwannoma (*red star*).

Box 3
Diagnostic criteria for neurofibromatosis type 2

A. Bilateral vestibular schwannomas or

B. First-degree relative with NF-2 and 1 of the following:
 • Unilateral vestibular schwannomas
 • Any 2 of the following:
  ○ Meningioma
  ○ Glioma
  ○ Schwannoma
  ○ Juvenile posterior lenticular opacities

Ref for table.[51]

---

presentation is multiple flat, light-brown patches of skin pigment (café-au-lait spots), skinfold freckling, visible neurofibromas under the skin, and small nodules of the iris (Lisch nodule). NF-1 is inherited in autosomal dominant fashion; however, 50% of mutations are detected de novo. Patients with NF-1 have a decreased life expectancy by 15 years when compared with the general population. The NF-1 gene is located on chromosome 17 and encodes for *neurofibromin*, which is a protein produced in nerve cells, oligodendrocytes, and Schwann cells (**Box 2, Fig. 7**).

NF-2 is also inherited in an autosomal dominant pattern, and affected individuals have a predisposition to formation of multiple nerve tumors. NF-2 is less common than NF-1 with an incidence of 1 in 25,000 people. The associated mutation is located on a gene that produces the protein, merlin, on chromosome 22q12.[50,52] The average age of death is 36 years with a 10-year survival rate of 67%. Patients with NF-2 develop vestibular schwannomas, as well as neurogenic tumors on other cranial nerves, spinal roots, and peripheral nerves. These patients often develop multiple meningiomas and ependymomas at an early age. Symptoms include hearing loss, balance problem, flesh-colored skin flaps, and muscle wasting. There are ongoing clinical trials to evaluate the role of bevacizumab for the treatment of patients with NF-2[51] (**Box 3**).

Box 4
Diagnostic criteria for schwannomatosis

Definite schwannomatosis
• Age greater than 30 years and 2 or more noncutaneous schwannomas (at least 1 with histologic confirmation) with no evidence of vestibular tumor on brain MRI scan and no known NF mutation
• Nonvestibular schwannoma (pathologically confirmed) plus first-degree relative who meets criteria of schwannomatosis

Possible schwannomatosis
• Age less than 30 years plus 2 or more noncutaneous schwannomas (at least 1 with histologic confirmation) with no evidence of vestibular tumor on brain MRI scan and no known NF mutation
• Age greater than 45 years plus 2 or more noncutaneous schwannomas (at least 1 with histologic confirmation) and no symptoms of eighth nerve dysfunction and NF-2
• Evidence of a nonvestibular schwannoma and first-degree relative meeting criteria for definite schwannomatosis

Ref for table.[51]

Schwannomatosis is the rarest form of NF and presents as multiple schwannomas in the absence of vestibular schwannomas. Schwannomatosis is also inherited in an autosomal dominant pattern with an incidence of 1 in 40,000 to 1 in 1.7 million people. Patients with schwannomatosis have a normal life expectancy, diagnosed at a median age of 40 years. The most common symptom is pain[51] (**Box 4**).

Surgery is a treatment of clinically symptomatic schwannomas and neurofibromas in patients affected by NF-1. However, recurrences are not uncommon following neurofibroma excision, especially plexiform neurofibromas. Surgery does not play a role in NF-2, unless patients are symptomatic from brainstem compression, hearing loss, or facial nerve dysfunction. More targeted therapies are currently under investigation.

CLINICS CARE POINTS

- Benign neurogenic tumors can grow and cause compression of structures, and also have potential for malignant transformation. Therefore, surgical resection is recommended.
- CT and/or MRI should be considered for preoperative planning.

DISCLOSURE

The authors have nothing to disclose.

REFERENCES

1. Kransdorf MJ. Benign soft-tissue tumors in a large referral population: distribution of specific diagnoses by age, sex, and location. AJR Am J Roentgenol 1995; 164(2):395–402.
2. Rha SE, Byun JY, Jung SE, et al. Neurogenic tumors in the abdomen: tumor types and imaging characteristics. Radiographics 2003;23(1):29–43.
3. Galetta D, Spaggiari L. Primary intrathoracic neurogenic tumors: clinical, pathological, and long-term outcomes. Thorac Cardiovasc Surg 2021;69(8): 749–55.
4. Kim DH, Murovic JA, Tiel RL, et al. Operative outcomes of 546 Louisiana State University Health Sciences Center peripheral nerve tumors. Neurosurg Clin N Am 2004;15(2):177–92.
5. Abreu E, Aubert S, Wavreille G, et al. Peripheral tumor and tumor-like neurogenic lesions. Eur J Radiol 2013;82(1):38–50.
6. Tagliafico AS, Isaac A, Bignotti B, et al. Nerve Tumors: What the MSK Radiologist Should Know. Semin Musculoskelet Radiol 2019;23(1):76–84.
7. Shimada H, Ambros IM, Dehner LP, et al. The International Neuroblastoma Pathology Classification (the Shimada system). Cancer 1999;86(2):364–72.
8. Lonergan GJ, Schwab CM, Suarez ES, et al. Neuroblastoma, ganglioneuroblastoma, and ganglioneuroma: radiologic-pathologic correlation. Radiographics 2002;22(4):911–34.
9. Maris JM. Recent advances in neuroblastoma. N Engl J Med 2010;362(23): 2202–11.
10. Spinelli C, Rossi L, Barbetta A, et al. Incidental ganglioneuromas: a presentation of 14 surgical cases and literature review. J Endocrinol Invest 2015;38(5):547–54.
11. Fliedner SMJ, Winkelmann PER, Wesley R, et al. Ganglioneuromas across age groups: Systematic review of individual patient data. Clin Endocrinol (Oxf) 2021;94(1):12–23.

12. Sandru F, Dumitrascu MC, Petca A, et al. Adrenal ganglioneuroma: Prognostic factors (Review). Exp Ther Med 2021;22(5):1338.
13. Fassnacht M, Arlt W, Bancos I, et al. Management of adrenal incidentalomas: European Society of Endocrinology Clinical Practice Guideline in collaboration with the European Network for the Study of Adrenal Tumors. Eur J Endocrinol 2016; 175(2):G1–34.
14. Thompson LD. Pheochromocytoma of the Adrenal gland Scaled Score (PASS) to separate benign from malignant neoplasms: a clinicopathologic and immunophenotypic study of 100 cases. Am J Surg Pathol 2002;26(5):551–66.
15. Lenders JW, Duh Q, Eisenhofer G, et al. Pheochromocytoma and paraganglioma: an endocrine society clinical practice guideline. J Clin Endocrinol Metab 2014; 99(6):1915–42.
16. Gannan E, van Veenendaal P, Scarlett A, et al. Retroperitoneal non-functioning paraganglioma: A difficult tumour to diagnose and treat. Int J Surg Case Rep 2015;17:133–5.
17. Feng N, Zhang WY, Wu XT. Clinicopathological analysis of paraganglioma with literature review. World J Gastroenterol 2009;15(24):3003–8.
18. Tischler AS, Kimura N, McNicol AM. Pathology of pheochromocytoma and extra-adrenal paraganglioma. Ann N Y Acad Sci 2006;1073:557–70.
19. Somasundar P, Krouse R, Hostetter R, et al. Paragangliomas– a decade of clinical experience. J Surg Oncol 2000;74(4):286–90.
20. Isik AC, Imamoglu M, Erem C, et al. Paragangliomas of the head and neck. Med Princ Pract 2007;16(3):209–14.
21. Leung AA, Pasieka JL, Hyrcza MD, et al. Epidemiology of pheochromocytoma and paraganglioma: population-based cohort study. Eur J Endocrinol 2021; 184(1):19–28.
22. Fishbein L, Merrill S, Fraker DL, et al. Inherited mutations in pheochromocytoma and paraganglioma: why all patients should be offered genetic testing. Ann Surg Oncol 2013;20(5):1444–50.
23. Hamidi O, Young WF, Iniguez-Ariza NM, et al. Malignant Pheochromocytoma and Paraganglioma: 272 Patients Over 55 Years. J Clin Endocrinol Metab 2017; 102(9):3296–305.
24. Cascon A, Pita G, Burnichon N, et al. Genetics of pheochromocytoma and paraganglioma in Spanish patients. J Clin Endocrinol Metab 2009;94(5): 1701–5.
25. Fishbein L, Del Rivero J, Else T, et al. The North American Neuroendocrine Tumor Society Consensus Guidelines for Surveillance and Management of Metastatic and/or Unresectable Pheochromocytoma and Paraganglioma. Pancreas 2021; 50(4):469–93.
26. Lenders JW, Eisenhofer G, Mannelli M, et al. Phaeochromocytoma. Lancet 2005; 366(9486):665–75.
27. Mannelli M, Ianni L, Cilotti A, et al. Pheochromocytoma in Italy: a multicentric retrospective study. Eur J Endocrinol 1999;141(6):619–24.
28. Harari A, Inabnet WB 3rd. Malignant pheochromocytoma: a review. Am J Surg 2011;201(5):700–8.
29. Goldstein RE, O'Neill JA, Holcomb GW, et al. Clinical experience over 48 years with pheochromocytoma. Ann Surg 1999;229(6):755–64 [discussion: 764-766].
30. Goffredo P, Sosa JA, Roman SA. Malignant pheochromocytoma and paraganglioma: a population level analysis of long-term survival over two decades. J Surg Oncol 2013;107(6):659–64.

31. Hescot S, Curras-Freixes M, Deutschbein T, et al. Prognosis of Malignant Pheochromocytoma and Paraganglioma (MAPP-Prono Study): A European Network for the Study of Adrenal Tumors Retrospective Study. J Clin Endocrinol Metab 2019;104(6):2367–74.

32. Kimura N, Takayanagi R, Takizawa N, et al. Pathological grading for predicting metastasis in phaeochromocytoma and paraganglioma. Endocr Relat Cancer 2014;21(3):405–14.

33. Werbel SS, Ober KP. Pheochromocytoma. Update on diagnosis, localization, and management. Med Clin North Am 1995;79(1):131–53.

34. Eisenhofer G, Goldstein DS, Sullivan P, et al. Biochemical and clinical manifestations of dopamine-producing paragangliomas: utility of plasma methoxytyramine. J Clin Endocrinol Metab 2005;90(4):2068–75.

35. Brouwers FM, Lenders JW, Eisenhofer G, et al. Pheochromocytoma as an endocrine emergency. Rev Endocr Metab Disord 2003;4(2):121–8.

36. Neumann HPH, Young WF Jr, Eng C. Pheochromocytoma and Paraganglioma. N Engl J Med 2019;381(6):552–65.

37. Sjoberg RJ, Simcic KJ, Kidd GS. The clonidine suppression test for pheochromocytoma. A review of its utility and pitfalls. Arch Intern Med 1992;152(6):1193–7.

38. Archier A, Varoquaux A, Garrigue P, et al. Prospective comparison of (68)Ga-DOTATATE and (18)F-FDOPA PET/CT in patients with various pheochromocytomas and paragangliomas with emphasis on sporadic cases. Eur J Nucl Med Mol Imaging 2016;43(7):1248–57.

39. Fang F, Ding L, He Q, et al. Preoperative management of pheochromocytoma and paraganglioma. Front Endocrinol (Lausanne) 2020;11:586795.

40. Kercher KW, Novitsky YW, Park A, et al. Laparoscopic curative resection of pheochromocytomas. Ann Surg 2005;241(6):919–26 [discussion: 926-928].

41. Fu SQ, Wang SY, Chen Q, et al. Laparoscopic versus open surgery for pheochromocytoma: a meta-analysis. BMC Surg 2020;20(1):167.

42. Aliyev S, Karabulut K, Agcaoglu O, et al. Robotic versus laparoscopic adrenalectomy for pheochromocytoma. Ann Surg Oncol 2013;20(13):4190–4.

43. Araujo-Castro M, Centero RG, Lopez-Garcia MC, et al. Surgical outcomes in the pheochromocytoma surgery. Results from the PHEO-RISK STUDY. Endocrine 2021;74(3):676–84.

44. Pryma DA, Chin BB, Noto RB, et al. Efficacy and Safety of High-Specific-Activity (131)I-MIBG Therapy in Patients with Advanced Pheochromocytoma or Paraganglioma. J Nucl Med 2019;60(5):623–30.

45. Ayala-Ramirez M, Feng L, Habra MA, et al. Clinical benefits of systemic chemotherapy for patients with metastatic pheochromocytomas or sympathetic extraadrenal paragangliomas: insights from the largest single-institutional experience. Cancer 2012;118(11):2804–12.

46. Patel D, Phay JE, Yen TWF, et al. Update on Pheochromocytoma and Paraganglioma from the SSO Endocrine and Head and Neck Disease Site Working Group, Part 2 of 2: Perioperative Management and Outcomes of Pheochromocytoma and Paraganglioma. Ann Surg Oncol 2020;27(5):1338–47.

47. Fallon M, Tadi P. Histology, Schwann cells. Treasure Island (FL: StatPearls; 2022.

48. Goh BK, Tan Y, Chung YA, et al. Retroperitoneal schwannoma. Am J Surg 2006; 192(1):14–8.

49. Murphey MD, Smith WS, Smith SE, et al. From the archives of the AFIP. Imaging of musculoskeletal neurogenic tumors: radiologic-pathologic correlation. Radiographics 1999;19(5):1253–80.

50. Hilton DA, Hanemann CO. Schwannomas and their pathogenesis. Brain Pathol 2014;24(3):205–20.
51. Tamura R. Current Understanding of Neurofibromatosis Type 1, 2, and Schwannomatosis. Int J Mol Sci 2021;22(11):5850.
52. Rouleau GA, Merel P, Lutchman M, et al. Alteration in a new gene encoding a putative membrane-organizing protein causes neuro-fibromatosis type 2. Nature 1993;363(6429):515–21.